Body Fitness and Exercise

SECOND EDITION

Basic theory and practice for therapists

Body Fitness and Exercise

SECOND EDITION

Basic theory and practice for therapists

Mo Rosser

Hodder & Stoughton

A MEMBER OF THE HODDER HEADLINE GROUP

British Library Cataloguing in Publication Data

ISBN 0 340 789565

Second edition 2001
First published 1995
Impression number   10 9 8 7 6 5 4 3 2 1
Year   2005 2004 2003 2002 2001

Typeset by Servis Filmsetting Ltd
Printed in Great Britain for Hodder & Stoughton Educational, a division
of Hodder Headline Plc, 338 Euston Road, London NW1 3BH
by Martins the Printers Ltd, Spittal, Berwick upon Tweed

Contents

Er Côf am rhieni annwyl
William Aldwyn a Catherine Read

Acknowledgements

I am indebted to many people for their advice and support during the preparation of this book. In particular, my thanks to Sue Wandless for reading and advising on the text. For their encouragement and patience, I thank Elsie Rosser, Sue Rosser and Helen Price, and my husband, Gwyn, for his consistent support. Special thanks also to Suzie Robertson and Jeff Rosser, who meticulously typed, prepared and organised the manuscript.

The author and publisher would like to thank the following, for permission and assistance in the reproduction of copyright photographs and material: Accoson Ltd, fig. 10.5; British Medical Association, fig. 10.4; Pharma Plast Ltd, fig. 8.2; Powersport International Ltd, fig. 8.5 & p. 91; Ragdale Hall Health Hydro, fig. 10.1 & p. 135; Vitalograph Ltd, fig. 10.3. Permission has been granted by the publisher, Edward Arnold, for the reproduction of several figures from: Sears, W. Gordon (1985) *Anatomy and Physiology for Nurses*, eds. R. S. Winwood and E. Sears, London: Edward Arnold (figs. 2.8, 3.4–3.17, 3.19, 3.21, 4.6, 5.1, 5.2, 5.4).

Every effort has been made to obtain permission for the reproduction of copyright material. Any queries regarding such should be addressed to the publisher.

Photographs on pages 1, 139, 145, 148, 257 appear courtesy of Action Plus.

Cover photograph appears courtesy of The Stock Market, London.

PART A

Underpinning Knowledge Anatomical, Physiological and Physical Concepts

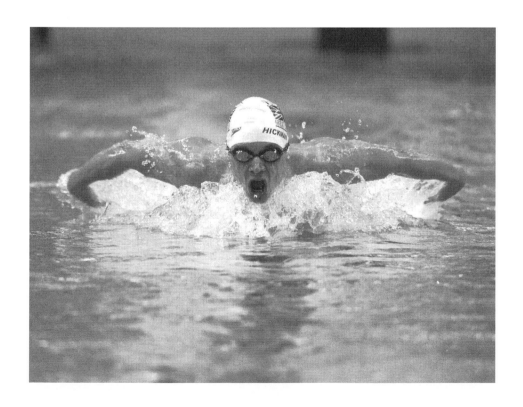

Introduction

Regular exercise will produce beneficial effects for any age group providing the exercise is specific and appropriate to the level of fitness of the individual. Progressive exercise, correctly performed will increase the level of fitness and improve health. It will also create a sense of well-being, produce greater energy and reduce the risk of developing many diseases. Exercise makes demands on the body systems over and above normal everyday activities and as a result the systems adapt anatomically and physiologically. All activities involve the co-ordinated interaction of many body systems. The muscular system and the skeletal system interact to produce movement, the contracting muscles exert a force or pull on the bones, resulting in movement at the joints. Muscle contraction requires energy, which is supplied by nutrients from the digestive system and oxygen from the respiratory system. These products are delivered to the muscles by the cardio-vascular system which also transports the waste products of metabolism such as carbon dioxide and lactic acid away from the contracting muscles. The nervous system and endocrine system are also involved with the control and regulation of movement.

These systems will cope efficiently with everyday activities as they are physiologically adapted to that level. However, if the activities suddenly increase, the systems are stressed and are initially unable to cope with the extra demand. But if the higher level of activity is maintained over a period of time, the systems gradually adapt and improve until they are able to cope efficiently again. This is the fundamental principle of training, i.e. gradually increasing the stress or demand on the systems in order to produce physiological adaptation and improvement.

You will be familiar with the symptoms felt when the body systems are over stressed, e.g. suddenly running for a bus will produce breathlessness and panting: the first sporting event of the season will produce muscle soreness. However if these activities are repeated on a regular basis these symptoms diminish with time because certain physiological adaptations and improvements have taken place enabling the systems to function more efficiently.

Training programmes may be adapted and tailored to meet the needs of a specific sport or athletic performance, e.g weight training to improve muscle strength for weight lifters or aerobic training to improve endurance for distance runners.

It is important to remember that beneficial effects are only derived from exercise that is appropriate, progressive and correctly performed. Inappropriate exercise, casually performed, may result in injury, pain and stiffness.

Teachers of exercise have to be aware of their responsibility for the safety of those in their care. They are educators, advisers and role models and therefore require sufficient knowledge to deliver safe and effective exercise and to give accurate advice.

This book covers the basic theory of fitness and exercise and will enable the student to construct suitable programmes to meet a variety of needs. It is impossible to cover all types of exercise in one book and further reading about specific training regimes is required. Students must keep abreast of new developments and use knowledge carefully for the benefit of their clients.

To fully understand how the body benefits from exercise it is important to have a basic understanding of body structure and function. The following chapters will provide you with a basic knowledge of anatomy and physiology and how the systems interact and adapt as a result of exercise.

Chapter 1
Organisational levels

To appreciate fully the effects of exercise and to educate their clients, all exercise therapists must have a sound basic knowledge of anatomy and physiology.

- Anatomy is the study of the structure of the body.
- Physiology is the study of the functions of the body

The structure of each system is adapted and designed to carry out certain specific functions. The systems interact with each other in a co-ordinated manner to maintain the stable internal environment required by cells for proper functioning. The maintenance of a stable internal environment is known as *homeostasis*. An in-depth study of these subjects is not within the scope of this book and the therapist should refer to a specialist anatomy and physiology textbook.

This first section will review the body systems and elaborate specifically on those involved in movement, namely the skeletal and muscular systems.

THE ORGANISATIONAL LEVELS OF THE BODY

Chemical → Cellular → Tissue → Organ → Body System

CHEMICAL

At the very basic level, we have the chemical elements which form the body mass and are essential for maintaining life. Reactions in which these chemicals are combined or broken down underlie all the processes necessary for sustaining life.

CELLULAR

The cells are the basic structural and functional units of the body. All the activities that maintain life are carried out by the cells. The body is made up of billions of cells: they all have a similar basic structure, but change slightly to suit their function, for example blood cells differ from fat cells.

Cells are bathed in extracellular fluid; this provides a medium for the exchange of nutrients and oxygen from the capillary blood into the cells and the removal of the waste products of metabolism from the cells into the capillary blood.

The structure of a typical cell

The cell membrane or plasma membrane
This is the outer layer or boundary of the cell. It gives shape to the cell and protects it, separating things inside the cell (intracellular) from those outside the cell (extracellular). It regulates the passage of substances in and out of the cell.

The cytoplasm
This is a soft, jelly-like substance where the functions of the cell are carried out. It contains various structures called organelles (mini-organs), each of which has a specific function. Also in the cytoplasm are various chemical substances called inclusions.

The organelles
These mini-organs each have a characteristic shape and a specific role to perform. The type and number of organelles in different kinds of cells vary depending on the activities of the cell; for example, muscle cells have large numbers of mitochondria, because they have a high level of energy output.

- The largest of the organelles is the nucleus. It controls the activities of the cell and it contains the body's genetic material (DNA).

Other organelles include:

- Mitochondria, which generate ATP/energy; there are large numbers in muscle cells;
- Ribosomes, which synthesise protein;
- Lysosomes, which digest and deal with waste;
- The Golgi apparatus which is concerned with the production of membrane and protein lipids and glycoproteins;
- Endoplasmic reticulum – a series of channels for transporting substances within the cell;
- The centrosome, involved in cell division.

The inclusions
These are chemical substances produced by cells. They may not be present in all cells. For example, melanin is a pigment found in certain cells of the skin and hair; it protects the body by

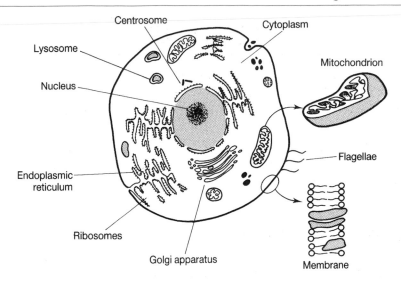

FIGURE NUMBER: 1.1 – A typical cell.

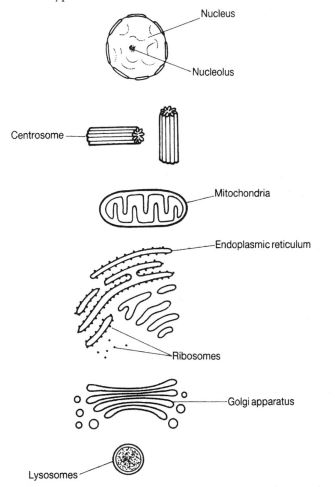

FIGURE NUMBER: 1.2 – Organelles found in the cell.

screening out ultra-violet light, and gives the skin its brown colour on exposure to sunlight. Lipids (fat) is found in fat cells; this is broken down to provide energy when required.

The characteristics of cells

All living things, whether they be single-celled or multi-celled organisms, have certain characteristics or functions in common that are essential to life:

Metabolism

This is the sum total of all the cells' chemical activities. There are two phases of metabolism:

- *Catabolism* is the breaking down of chemical substances derived from food to provide the energy and heat needed to sustain life;
- *Anabolism* uses the energy of catabolism to build new chemical compounds and repair tissues.

Respiration

This involves two processes – external respiration: the movement of gases in and out of the lungs and circulating blood, and internal respiration: the metabolic activities within the cells.

Cells are capable of producing energy from food substances taken in by or stored in the body. When oxygen is utilised in this process, it is termed *aerobic respiration*; when oxygen is not utilised in the process, it is termed *anaerobic respiration*.

Growth

Cells grow in size up to a certain limit. When this limit is reached the cells divide.

Reproduction

When the growth of cells is complete, they divide to produce two daughter cells that are identical to each other. This process of cell division is known as *mitosis*.

Excretion

Cells are capable of getting rid of the waste products resulting from metabolism; these pass out of the cell through the cell membrane into the tissue fluid, they then pass through capillary walls into the circulating blood.

Irritability

Cells are capable of responding to stimuli, which may be physical, chemical or thermal.

Movement

Some cells are capable of movement. They move by pushing out fingers of cytoplasm called pseudopodia or by the movement of flagellae.

The body is made up of billions of cells; they are similar in structure but not exactly the same, as they are modified (changed) to carry out specific functions. All the metabolic functions necessary for sustaining life are carried out by the cells.

The energy for the metabolic activities of each cell is derived from the breakdown of a particular chemical compound – adenosine triphosphate, or ATP. Only a small amount of ATP is stored in the cells; once this is used up it must be continually resynthesised (produced). The production of ATP is a continuous process and comes from the energy released from certain high energy chemicals and the breakdown of the foods we eat, mainly the carbohydrates and fats. Muscle cells expend far more energy (for muscle contraction) than other cells and must be able to continually resynthesise large amounts of ATP/Energy.

Three metabolic systems contribute to this energy production: the phosphagen system, anaerobic glycolysis, and the aerobic system. These are discussed in chapter 4.

Summary and aid to learning

The body is made up of billions of cells similar in structure but not identical as they are modified to carry out specific functions. All the metabolic functions necessary for sustaining life are carried out by the cells.

Cells are composed of *cytoplasm*, containing *organelles* which is surrounded and contained by the *cell membrane*.

The *nucleus* is the largest organelle; it controls all the functions carried out by the cell and contains the body's genetic material or DNA.

Each organelle has a specific, life-sustaining role to play.

The energy for the metabolic activities of every cell is derived from the breakdown of a particular chemical compound – adenosine triphosphate, or ATP.

Mitochondria produce ATP; they produce the energy for all the activities of the cell and consequently are known as powerhouses or power plants.

Only a small amount of ATP is stored in the cells; once this is used up it must be continually resynthesised (produced).

The production of ATP is a continuous process and comes from the energy released from certain high energy chemical compounds and the breakdown of the foods we eat, mainly carbohydrates and fats.

LEARN

Characteristics or functions of cells:

- Metabolism
- Respiration
- Growth
- Reproduction
- Excretion
- Irritability
- Movement

TISSUES

The tissues of the body are made up of groups of similar cells that work together to perform a specific function. All the cells of one tissue will be identical, but the cells of different tissues will be modified to suit tissue function. There are four main types of tissue in the body:

- *Epithelial tissue* covers the body's surfaces, lines the organs and tubes and forms glands;
- *Connective tissue* supports and protects organs, binds and connects tissues and organs together and provides storage of fat for energy reserves;
- *Muscle tissue* is able to contract and relax to produce movement;
- *Nervous tissue* initiates and transmits impulses to co-ordinate the activities of the body. It is the communication system of the body.

Epithelial tissue or epithelium

This tissue forms the outer covering of body surfaces and body organs. It also forms the inner lining of organs, tracts, vessels and ducts. Glandular epithelium lines glands and secretes substances.

Epithelium is composed of closely packed cells. There are two main classifications:

- simple epithelium, which is a single layer of cells;
- stratified or compound epithelium, which consists of many layers of cells.

It may be further sub-classified according to the shape of the cells. The many types of epithelium may be summarised as shown in Tables 1.1 and 1.2.

Table 1.1
Types of simple epithelium

Name	Type	Location
Squamous (a)	flat cells	lines heart and blood vessels, alveoli
Cuboidal (b)	cube-shaped cells	lines kidney tubules, ducts of glands
Columnar (c)	cells like columns	lines stomach and digestive tract
Columnar ciliated (d)	columns with hair-like cilia	lines respiratory tract and fallopian tubes

These chemicals regulate certain physiological processes.

Glandular epithelium contains cells that secrete substances and is found in glands.

- Exocrine glands secrete substances into ducts or directly onto surfaces: for example, sweat glands secrete sweat, salivary glands secrete saliva and various digestive tract glands secrete digestive juices.

■ Endocrine glands, for example the adrenal and thyroid glands, secrete hormones directly into the blood.

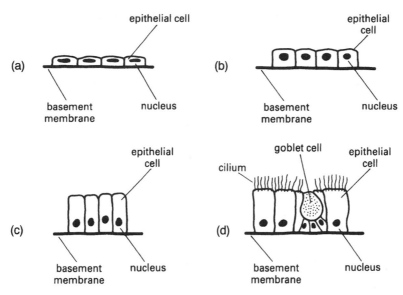

FIGURE NUMBER: 1.3 – Simple epithelium.

Table 1.2
Types of compound epithelium

Name	Type	Location
Squamous (a)	layers of flat cells	non-keratinised: lines mouth, tongue, oesophagus
		keratinised: forms outer layer of skin
Cuboidal (b)	layers of flat cube-shaped cells	ducts of sweat glands
Columnar (c)	layers of columnar cells	lines parts of male urethra, anus
Transitional (d & e)	layers of cells which compress and allow tissues to be distended	lines bladder, ureters and urethra

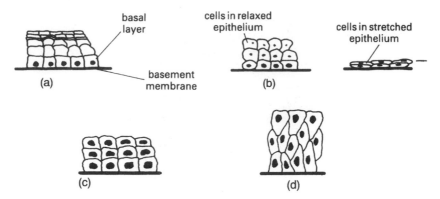

FIGURE NUMBER: 1.4 – Compound of epithelium.

Connective tissue

This is the most widely distributed tissue in the body. There are many different types of connective tissue, all with specific functions. Connective tissue is composed of a ground substance or matrix. in which are found widely scattered cells and fibres. The type of matrix or intercellular substance determines the type of connective tissue; for example, some types of tissue are fluid, some are soft and some are firm and flexible, while others are hard and rigid. The general functions of connective tissue are protection, support, the connection or joining together of various structures and the separation of others, and the storage of energy reserves.

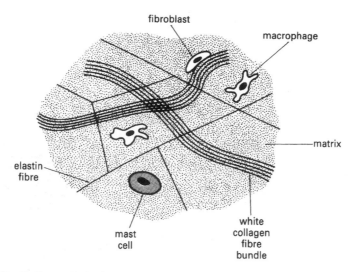

FIGURE NUMBER: 1.5 – Areolar tissue.

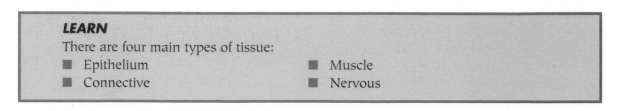

> *LEARN*
> There are four main types of tissue:
> - Epithelium
> - Connective
> - Muscle
> - Nervous

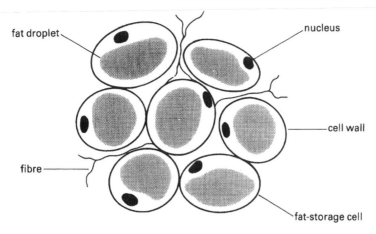

FIGURE NUMBER: 1.6 – Adipose tissue.

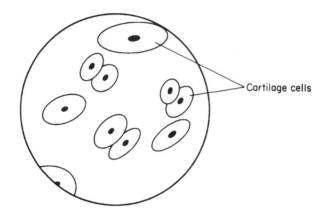

FIGURE NUMBER: 1.7 – Hyaline cartilage.

Table 1.3 Types of connective tissue		
Name	*Structure*	*Location/function*
Areolar tissue	loose moist tissue with a viscous matrix and a loose, irregular arrangement of fibres: white fibres for strength and yellow fibres for elasticity. A variety of cells are found scattered throughout	widely distributed as dermis of skin and under the skin as superficial fascia; found between muscles and other tissues and around organs. It gives strength, elasticity and support

[continued]

Name	Structure	Location/function
Adipose tissue	loose connective tissue, with large numbers of specialised cells, called *adipocytes*, for fat storage. The cytoplasm and nucleus of the cell are pushed to one side and fat fills the cell	subcutaneous layer of skin, the amount varying between thin and obese people; around heart and kidney; in the marrow of long bones; as padding around joints. Regular aerobic exercise will utilise the fats from these stores as a source of energy
Dense or white fibrous connective tissue	composed of closely packed bundles of fibres, mainly white collagen fibres, interspersed with cells	forms tendons and aponeuroses that attach muscle to bone, and ligaments that hold bones together; provides a protective covering for organs, e.g. kidney, heart, liver, testes
Yellow elastic tissue	composed mainly of yellow elastic fibres with few fibroblasts. This tissue gives elasticity and strength, recoiling to its original shape after stretching	forms the walls of arteries, trachea, bronchial tubes and the lungs. It allows organs to stretch and recoil
Reticular tissue	reticular fibres form a delicate network with cells wrapped around them	forms delicate support in organs such as spleen, lymph nodes, liver
Cartilage (three types) *hyaline cartilage*	consists of a gelatinous intercellular matrix with fine collagen fibres and cells called *chondrocytes*. Hyaline cartilage is smooth, tough, resilient and flexible. It is milky white with a bluish tinge. It is commonly called gristle	covers the ends or articulating surfaces of bones; forms the costal cartilages, the rings of the trachea and bronchi and the nasal septum; provides a smooth surface to minimise friction at joints. With age, injury or disease this cartilage may be damaged or eroded, and friction at the joint increases as bone rubs on bone, producing pain and stiffness

[continued]

Name	Structure	Location/function
fibro-cartilage	similar to hyaline, but the matrix contains bundles of collagen fibres with widely dispersed chondrocytes. The fibres give strength, toughness and flexibility. It gives a slight cushioning effect when compressed	found in the symphysis pubis, inter-vertebral discs and the menisci of the knee. It supports and cushions. Severe compression and abnormal movements can damage discs and menisci. These are common injuries in sport and exercise (see chapter 3)
elastic cartilage	similar to hyaline, but the matrix consists of freely branching elastic fibres with dispersed chondrocytes. It is flexible and resilient. It gives support and shape	found in the epiglottis and external ear, giving shape and support
Bone or osseous tissue (two types)		
compact bone	hard, dense, ivory-like tissue	forms the outer layer of bones
cancellous bone	sponge-like structure with trabeculae and large spaces	found inside most bones
Blood	fluid connective tissue consisting of plasma and circulating cells	transports substances around the body. Regulates body heat. Prevents blood loss by coagulation

Summary and aid to learning

Each tissue of the body is composed of a mass of identical cells grouped together.

The cells of different tissues are basically the same but have changed slightly to suit their particular function.

There are four main tissue groups: Epithelium, connective, muscle, and nervous.

Each of these groups may be further subdivided. Read the text and list all the different types of cells found in each group.

Study the function of each type (see Table 1.3) and explain why the cells of adipose tissue differ from the cells of hyaline cartilage.

LEARN
Types of connective tissue:
- Areolar
- Adipose
- White fibrous
- Yellow elastic
- Reticular
- Cartilage
- Bone
- Blood

Muscle tissue

Muscle tissue is highly specialised, in that it is capable of contraction and relaxation. There are three types of muscle tissue:

- *Skeletal muscle* (voluntary; striated) forms the body flesh is attached to bones. When skeletal muscle contracts it pulls on the bones and produces movement at the joint. It also maintains posture and produces body heat. The cells of skeletal muscles are long cylindrical fibres with many nuclei (multi-nucleated); they have a striped or 'striated' appearance. These muscle fibres are arranged in bundles and many bundles group together to form a muscle. See chapter 6 for further detail.

- *Cardiac muscle* (involuntary; striated) forms the wall of the heart. When cardiac muscle contracts, the heart pumps blood around the body. The cells or fibres of cardiac muscles are quadrilateral in shape and contain only one nucleus. The cells branch, forming a network. The cells are separated from each other by thickened discs called intercalated discs.

- *Smooth muscle* (involuntary; non-striated) is found in the walls of blood vessels, the stomach, the intestine, the gall bladder and the urinary bladder. This muscle contracts to constrict blood vessels or to move food through the digestive tract and eliminate waste. The cells are spindle-shaped and contain a single nucleus. Moving food along the digestive tract is known as peristalsis. The constriction of blood vessels controls blood flow to an area. The narrowing of blood vessels reduces blood flow which can then be diverted to another area.

Summary and aid to learning

There are three types of muscle tissue: skeletal, cardiac and smooth. All three are able to contract and relax.

LEARN
Types of muscle tissue:
- Skeletal – body muscles
- Cardiac – heart
- Smooth – intestines, stomach

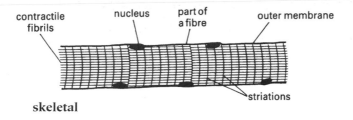

skeletal

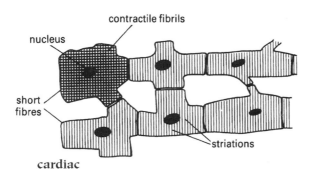

cardiac

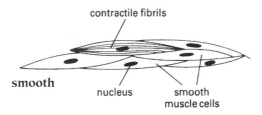

smooth

FIGURE NUMBER: 1.8 – Types of muscle tissue.

Skeletal muscle forms the body flesh and gives the body shape.

Skeletal muscle is known as *voluntary* because it is under the control of the will: we can decide if we want to move an arm or leg.

It is also known as *striated* because when looked at under a powerful microscope, stripes or striations can be seen across the length of the fibres.

The cells of skeletal muscle are long cylinder-like fibres with many nuclei.

When skeletal muscle contracts it pulls on bones which results in movement at the underlying joints.

Cardiac muscle is *striated* and found only in the walls of the heart.

Cardiac muscle is *involuntary* because it is not under the control of the will, we cannot control the contraction of the heart. This tissue is under the control of the autonomic nervous system.

The cells are quadrilateral in shape and contain one nucleus.

Smooth muscle is also *involuntary* and is under the control of the autonomic system.

It is *non–striated*, there are no stripes along its length.

The cells are spindle shaped with a single nucleus.

Smooth muscle is found in the walls of blood vessels, intestines, stomach etc.

Smooth muscle of the intestine contracts to move food along; this contraction and relaxation is known as *peristalsis*.

Smooth muscle also contracts to constrict blood vessels; this controls the blood flow to an area. When the vessels contract blood flow is reduced, when the vessels dilate more blood flows. Increased blood flow is an important factor during exercise when the contracting muscles depend on an increased delivery of nutrients and oxygen by the blood.

Nervous tissue

This tissue forms the nervous system; the body's communication system which initiates and controls body movement. It consists of two types of cells: *neurones* and *neuroglia*.

Neurones pick up stimuli and conduct impulses to other neurones, to muscle fibres or to glands. There are three types:
- *Motor neurones* conduct impulses from the brain and spinal cord to muscles and glands.
- *Sensory neurones* conduct impulses from the sensory organs to the brain and spinal cord.
- *Inter neurones* conduct impulses from one neurone to another.

Neuroglia support and protect neurones.

LEARN
Types of neurones:
- Motor neurones
- Sensory neurones
- Inter neurones

ORGANS

Many tissues combine to form the organs of the body. Each organ has a specific function or functions to perform.

For example, the stomach digests food, the lungs exchange gases, the heart pumps blood, the kidneys filter fluids and form urine, the ovaries produce and release ova. Organs combine to make up the systems of the body.

BODY SYSTEMS

Each body system consists of many organs that co-operate to perform various functions. All the systems are interrelated and function together to maintain life. There are eleven body systems, as shown in Table 1.4. During exercise and training the systems interact in a complex way to ensure optimum performance.

LEARN

The eleven body systems are:

- Integumentary
- Skeletal
- Muscular
- Nervous
- Cardio-vascular
- Lymphatic
- Respiratory
- Digestive
- Urinary
- Reproductive
- Endocrine

Table 1.4
The eleven body systems

System	Location	Function
Integumentary system	the skin and all its structures; nails; hair; sweat and sebaceous (oil) glands	protects; regulates temperature; eliminates waste; makes vitamin D; receives stimuli
Skeletal system	the bones, joints and cartilages	supports; protects; allows movement; stores fat and minerals; protects cells that produce blood cells

[continued]

System	Location	Function
Muscular system	usually refers to skeletal muscle, but includes cardiac and smooth muscle	produces movement; maintains posture; produces heat
Nervous system	brain; spinal cord; nerves; sense organs	communicates and co-ordinates body functions
Cardio-vascular system	heart; blood vessels; blood	transports substances around the body; helps regulate body temperature; prevents blood loss by blood clotting
Lymphatic system	lymphatic vessels, nodes, lymph ducts; spleen; tonsils; thymus gland	returns proteins and plasma to blood; carries fat from intestine to blood; filters body fluid, forms white blood cells, fights infection and protects against disease
Respiratory system	pharynx, larynx, trachea, bronchi and lungs	supplies oxygen and removes carbon dioxide
Digestive system	gastro-intestinal tract, i.e. mouth, pharynx, oesophagus, stomach, small intestine, large intestine, rectum, anus; salivary glands; gall bladder, liver and pancreas	physical and chemical breakdown of food; absorption of nutrients and elimination of waste
Urinary system	kidneys, ureters, bladder and urethra	helps to regulate chemical composition of blood; helps to balance the acid/alkali content of the body; eliminates urine
Reproductive system	Female: breasts, ovaries, uterus, uterine tubes, vagina, external genitalia Male: testes, epididymides, vas deferens, spermatic cords, seminal vesicles, ejaculatory ducts, prostate gland, penis	involved in reproduction and the production of sex hormones
Endocrine system	consists of ductless glands which produce and secrete hormones directly into the blood	hormones regulate a wide variety of body activities such as nutrition and growth, and they help maintain homeostasis

QUESTIONS

1. List the organisational levels of the body.
2. Give three functions of the cell membrane.
3. Name the organelles that carry out the following functions:
   a synthesise protein
   b deal with waste
   c generate energy.
4. Define the term *metabolism*, and name the two phases involved.
5. Complete the following sentences:
   … group together to form body tissues.
   Body systems are made up of many … .
6. List all the types of epithelial tissue and give the location of each.
7. a Name the tissue that stores body fat.
   b List three locations where fat is stored.
8. a List the three types of cartilage.
   b Name the cartilage that covers the articulating surfaces of bones.
9. Give the location of the following muscle tissues:
   a skeletal
   b smooth
   c cardiac.
   Draw a simple diagram of each tissue.
10. Name and give the function of the three types of neurone.

Chapter 2
The skeletal system

This chapter will help you to understand the structure and functions of bones, cartilages and joints.

- Bones form the framework of the body and act as levers.
- Cartilage protects the ends of bones allowing smooth movement and acts as a shock absorber.
- Joints are formed where two or more bones meet; this is where body movement takes place.

THE ANATOMICAL POSITION

Before we can describe body movement, we must have a basic position or static posture that is used as a common reference point for describing surfaces, relationships and directions of movement. This is known as the anatomical position.

Definition
In the *anatomical position*, the body is upright, with feet slightly apart and toes pointing forward. The arms hang at the sides with the palms of the hands facing forwards. (Note the difference from the normal relaxed standing position, where the palms of the hands face the sides of the body.)

With the body in this position the terminology related to structures and joint movement can be described.

Body planes
These are imaginary surfaces along which movements take place. There are three planes and they lie at right angles to each other:

- The *Sagittal Plane* lies parallel to the sagittal suture of the skull. This plane divides the body into right and left parts. The Median Sagittal divides the body into equal right and left parts;
- The *Coronal or Frontal Plane* lies parallel to the coronal suture of the skull. This plane divides the body into front and back;
- The *Horizontal or Transverse Plane* is parallel to a flat floor. This plane divides the body into upper and lower parts.

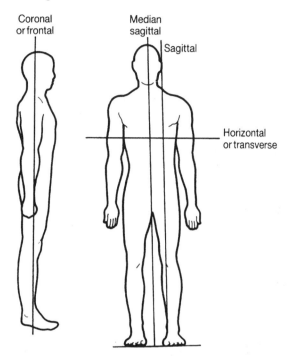

FIGURE NUMBER: 2.1 – Body planes.

LEARN

There are three planes:
- Sagittal
- Coronal (Frontal)
- Horizontal (Transverse)

Axes

The axis of a movement is a line around which the movement takes place (in the same way as a top spins about its axis). It is always at right angles to the plane of movement.

There are three axes of movement:
- *sagittal* – from back to front parallel to the sagittal suture of the skull;
- *coronal/frontal* – from side to side parallel to the coronal suture of the skull;
- *vertical* – straight up and down (vertical to the floor).

Examples of the planes and axes of certain movements when the body is in the anatomical position:

- flexion (bending) of the elbow is movement in a sagittal plane with a frontal axis;
- abduction of the hip (taking it out to the side) is movement in a frontal plane with a sagittal axis;
- turning the head from right to left is movement in a horizontal plane with a vertical axis.

LEARN

There are three axes:
- Sagittal
- Coronal (Frontal)
- Vertical

LEARN

Identify the plane of movement, then the axis will be at right angles to it.

TASK

Try the movements just described and work out others; remember that the movement must be in one of three planes and that the axis of the movement will be at right angles to that plane.

The functions of the skeletal system

- Support – the bony framework gives shape to the body, supports the soft tissues and provides attachment for muscles.
- Protection – the bony framework protects delicate internal organs from injury. For example, the brain is protected by the skull, the heart and lungs are protected by the rib cage.
- Movement – is produced by a system of bones, joints and muscles. The bones act as levers and muscles pull on the bones, resulting in movement at the joints.
- Storage of minerals – bones store many minerals, particularly calcium and phosphorus.
- Storage of energy – fats or lipids stored in the yellow bone marrow provide energy when required.
- Storage of tissue that forms blood cells – both red and white blood cells are produced by red bone marrow which is found in the spongy bone of the pelvis, vertebrae, ribs, sternum and in the ends of the femur and humerus.

LEARN

Functions of the skeletal system are:
- Support
- Protection
- Movement
- Storage of minerals, fats and tissue-forming blood cells

Terminology of surfaces and structures

It is important to be familiar with the terms used to describe surfaces of the body in the anatomical position and the position of structures relative to each other. These are shown in Figure 2.2 and described in Table 2.1.

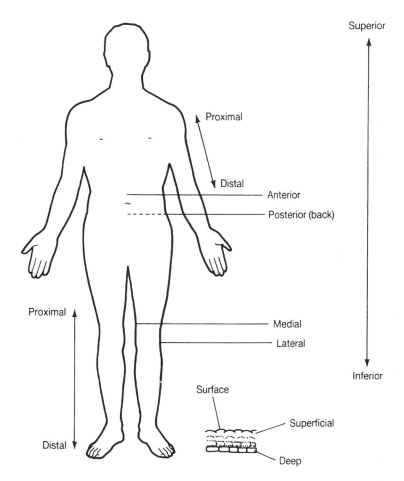

FIGURE NUMBER: 2.2 – Surfaces of the body.

The structure of bone

Bone is a very hard connective tissue consisting of cells, collagen fibres and a matrix or ground substance. The matrix is impregnated with mineral salts such as calcium carbonate and calcium phosphate. As these salts are laid down, the tissue calcifies and hardens. Bone is a flexible living tissue and has the capacity to repair if damaged. There are two types of bone tissue:

1 *Compact* bone is a hard dense tissue which forms the outer layer of bones and gives them strength.

2 *Cancellous* bone forms the inner mass of bone. The spongy structure makes bones lighter.

Table 2.1 Terminology used to describe the structure of the body	
Description of surface or structure	Position
Anterior or ventral	a surface that faces forwards; a structure that is further forwards than another
Posterior or dorsal	a surface that faces backwards; a structure that is further back than another
Medial	a surface or structure that is nearer to the mid-line than another
Lateral	a surface or structure that is further away from the mid-line than another
Proximal	a structure that is towards the root or origin, i.e. nearer the trunk
Distal	a structure that is further away from the root or origin, i.e. further away from the trunk
Superficial	a structure that is nearer the surface than others
Deep	a structure that lies beneath others, i.e. is further from the surface
Superior	a structure higher than others, i.e. nearer the head
Inferior	a structure lower than others, i.e. nearer the foot

Bones are enclosed in a dense layer of fibrous connective tissue known as the *periosteum*. This layer contains blood vessels which deliver nutrients to the bone, nerve and bone cells. Tendons (which attach muscles to bone) and ligaments (which join bones together) blend with the periosteum.

There are different types of *bone cells*, which are found in the periosteum or scattered throughout compact and spongy bone. They include:

■ *Osteoblasts*: the bone builders, which produce minerals and collagen needed for strong bones
■ *Osteocytes*: the main cells of bone tissue, which carry out the activities necessary for maintaining healthy bones
■ *Osteoclasts*: the bone clearers, which absorb and remove bone.

Exercise strengthens bones because they adapt to stress by laying down more calcium and other minerals, and also by increasing collagen fibres.

Fractures and other injuries to bones may occur in sports, and other physical activities. These must be quickly diagnosed and fixed to limit damage. An adequate length of time must be allowed for the fracture to heal.

> **LEARN**
> There are two types of bone tissue:
> - Compact bone – hard, dense. Forms the outer layer of bone for strength
> - Cancellous bone – spongy or honeycomb-like structure. Forms inner mass of bone for lightness

Types of bones forming the skeleton

There are four different types of bones named according to their shape:
- **Long bones** are longer than their width, e.g. femur, tibia, fibula, humerus, radius, ulna, metacarpals, phalanges.
- **Short bones** of almost equal width and length, e.g. carpal and tarsal bones.
- **Flat bones** are flat thin bones, found where protection is needed and also where a broad surface is required for the attachment of muscles, e.g. skull bones, scapulae, sternum, ribs.
- **Irregular bones** are all the bones with complex shapes that do not fit into the above categories, e.g. vertebrae, sacrum, innominate bone, sphenoid, ethmoid.

Other small bones found in the body but not named according to shape are called **sesamoid bones**: small rounded bones that develop within tendons, such as the patella. They enable the tendon to move smoothly over the underlying bone.

> **LEARN**
> The four types of bones forming the skeleton:
> - Long
> - Short
> - Flat
> - Irregular

Summary and aid to learning

Before we can describe anything relating to body structure and be understood by others we must use common reference points and terminology. We must refer to the body in the anatomical position.

Read the text and write a definition of the anatomical position; now stand or instruct a partner to stand in this position.

We also have words for describing surfaces and structures related to one another. These are best learnt as opposites:

anterior: towards the front	posterior: towards the back
proximal: nearer the body	distal: further away from the body
medial: towards mid-line	lateral: away from mid-line
superior: higher than another	inferior: lower than another
superficial: nearer the surface	deep: lies beneath another

Work with a partner and test each other by indicating to an aspect of the body which the other must identify.

The skeletal system includes the bones, joints and cartilages that make up the framework of the body.

The skeleton has specific functions. Read the text and explain the following:
- The skeleton gives the body a framework (how?)
- The skeleton protects (what?)
- The skeleton allows movement (how?)
- The skeleton stores (what and where?)

Bone is a connective tissue; a bone is composed of two different tissues:
- *Compact bone* which is dense, hard tissue and forms the outer covering of bones. It gives the bone its strength.
- *Cancellous bone* which is spongy or honeycomb-like in structure. It is light, making bones less heavy.

There are different types of bones which make up the skeleton. They are named according to their shape: long bones, short bones, flat bones and irregular bones. Can you give some examples of each type?

THE BONES OF THE SKELETON

It is difficult to study and visualise bones simply by using diagrams. It is easier to learn and much more interesting when a model skeleton and model bones are used. These can be examined and the important features identified and related to one's own body. Only the important and relevant features have been included in the following text. The bones are clearly labelled for easy learning. However, remember to identify the features on model bones and palpate (feel) on your own body where possible.

The human skeleton is made up of 206 bones. These are grouped into two main divisions: the *axial skeleton*, which forms the core or axis of the body, and the *appendicular skeleton*, which forms the girdles and limbs.

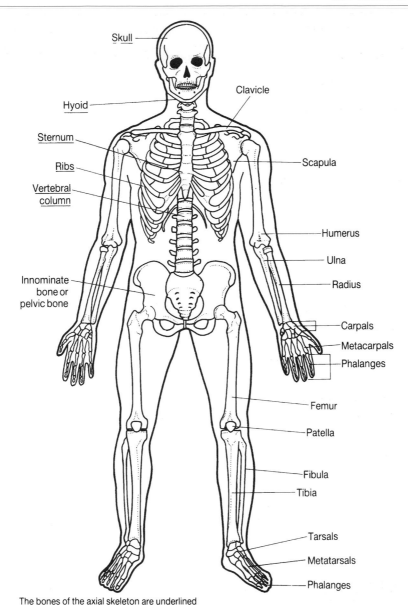

The bones of the axial skeleton are underlined

FIGURE NUMBER: 2.3 – The human skeleton.

The axial skeleton and the appendicular skeleton

The bones of the axial skeleton are the skull (head), the vertebral column (spine), the sternum (breast bone), the ribs, the hyoid bone (small bone in neck below mandible). The bones of the appendicular skeleton are as shown in Table 2.2.

Table 2.2 The bones of the appendicular skeleton	
Upper limb bones	*Lower limb bones*
Clavicle (collar bone)	Innominate/pelvic bone (hip bone)
Scapula (shoulder bone)	Femur (thigh bone)
Humerus (upper arm bone)	Patella (knee cap)
Radius (forearm – lateral)	Tibia (lower leg – medial)
Ulna (forearm – medial)	Fibula (lower leg – lateral)
Carpals (wrist)	Tarsals (ankle)
Metacarpals (palm)	Metatarsals (foot)
Phalanges (fingers)	Phalanges (toes)

The bones of the skull

These include the cranial and facial bones.

> **LEARN**
> There are eight cranial bones: one frontal, two parietal bones, one occipital, two temporal, one sphenoid and one ethmoid.
> In addition, there are fourteen facial bones; two lacrimal, two nasal bones, one vomer, two inferior nasal conchae or turbinate bones, two zygomatic bones, two palatine bones, two maxillae and one mandible.

The sutures of the skull

These are the joints between the bones of the skull. They are immovable fibrous joints. There are four main sutures: coronal, sagittal, lambdoidal and squamous.

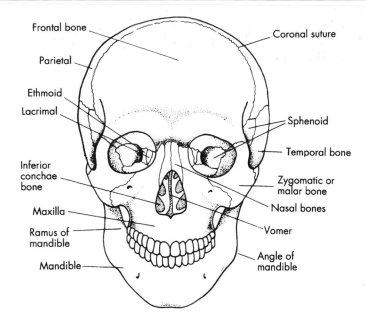

FIGURE NUMBER: 2.4 – The bones of the skull.

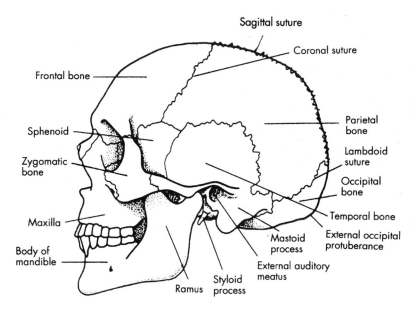

FIGURE NUMBER: 2.5 – Lateral view of the skull.

THE FEATURES OF THE SKELETAL BONES

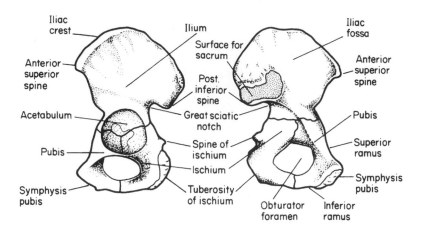

FIGURE NUMBER: 2.6 – The left innominate bone.

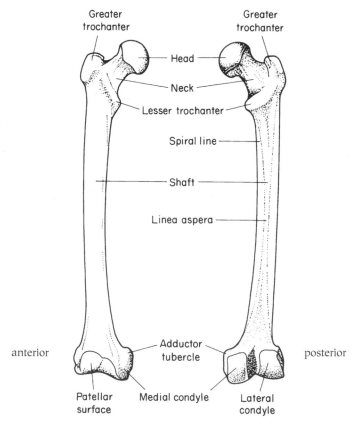

FIGURE NUMBER: 2.7 – Anterior and posterior views of the right femur.

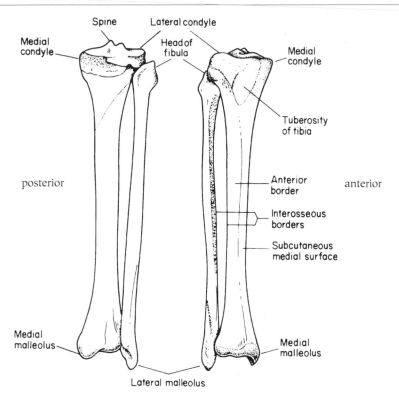

FIGURE NUMBER: 2.8 – Posterior and anterior views of the right tibia and fibula.

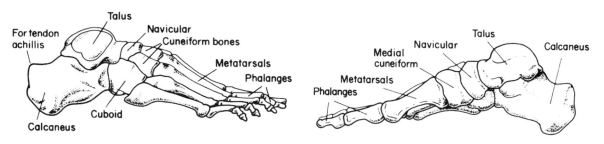

FIGURE NUMBER: 2.9 – The bones of the foot.

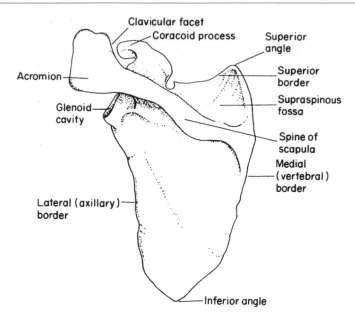

FIGURE NUMBER: 2.10 – The posterior surface of the scapula.

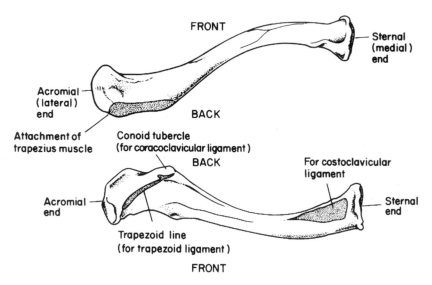

FIGURE NUMBER: 2.11 – The left clavicle.

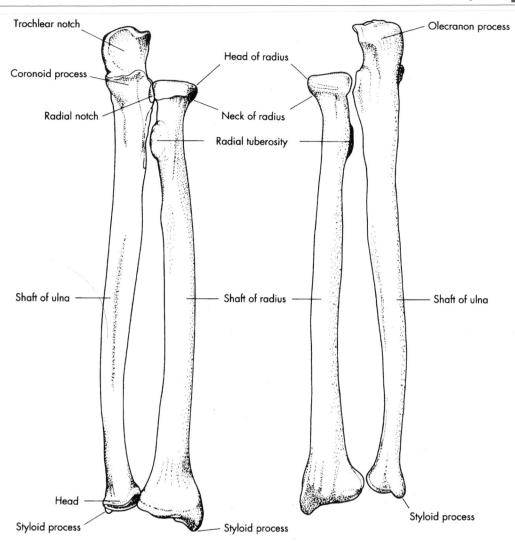

Trochlear notch

Coronoid process

Radial notch

Head of radius

Neck of radius

Radial tuberosity

Olecranon process

Shaft of ulna

Shaft of radius

Shaft of ulna

Head

Styloid process

Styloid process

Styloid process

FIGURE NUMBER: 2.12 – The left radius and ulna.

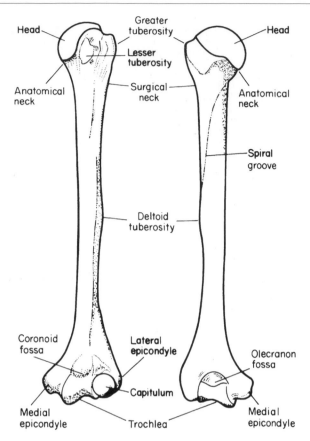

FIGURE NUMBER: 2.13 – The left humerus.

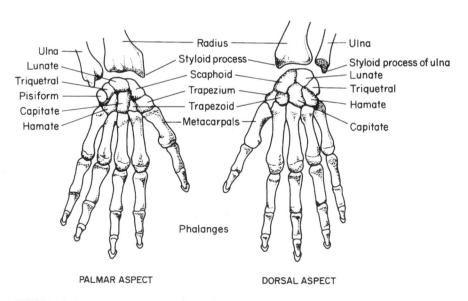

FIGURE NUMBER: 2.14 – The left hand.

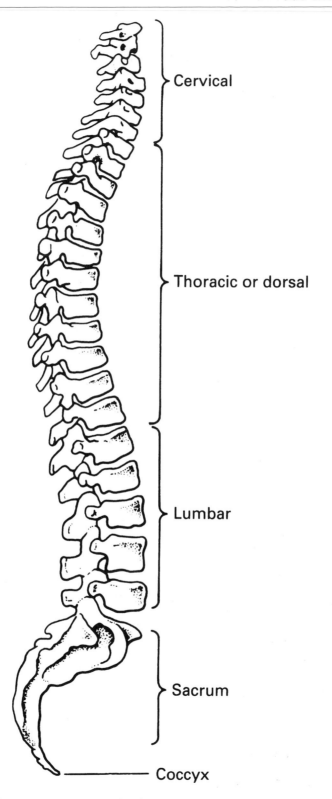

Cervical

Thoracic or dorsal

Lumbar

Sacrum

Coccyx

FIGURE NUMBER: 2.15 – The vertebral column.

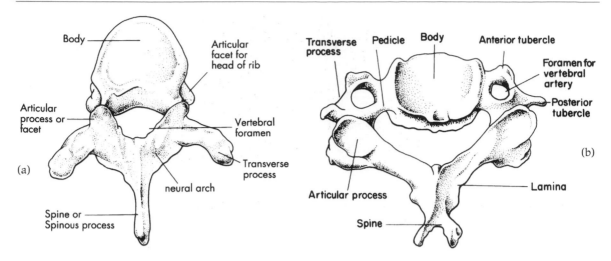

FIGURE NUMBER: 2.16 – (a) A thoracic vertebra. (b) A cervical vertebra.

The vertebral column (spinal column)

The vertebral column is composed of 33 vertebrae. Some are fused together, so that in fact there are only 26 bones. Between the bodies of adjacent vertebrae are discs of fibro cartilage which act as shock absorbers. These are called inter-vertebral discs. The column is divided into five regions:

- ■ *Cervical* – seven vertebrae (neck)
- ■ *Thoracic* – twelve vertebrae (upper back)
- ■ *Lumbar* – five vertebrae (small of back)
- ■ *Sacral* – five fused vertebrae (sacrum)
- ■ *Coccygeal* – four fused vertebrae (coccyx).

The functions of the vertebral column

- ■ It allows movement forward, backward and laterally.
- ■ It protects the spinal cord.
- ■ It supports the head.
- ■ It provides rigidity to maintain the upright posture.
- ■ It provides posterior attachment for the ribs.
- ■ It provides attachment for muscles.
- ■ It acts as a shock absorber due to the cushioning effect of the intervertebral discs.
- ■ The cancellous bone of the vertebrae stores red bone marrow, which forms blood cells.
- ■ It stores minerals.
- ■ It provides the fulcrum for numerous movements.

A typical vertebra

A typical vertebra is composed of several major parts:

- ■ the *body* – a mass of cancellous bone surrounded by a thin layer of compact bone. Body weight is transmitted through these bodies and the inter-vertebral discs that lie between them;

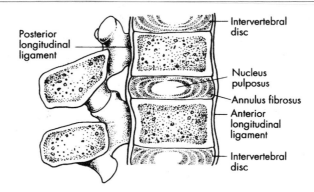

Posterior longitudinal ligament

Intervertebral disc

Nucleus pulposus

Annulus fibrosus

Anterior longitudinal ligament

Intervertebral disc

FIGURE NUMBER: 2.17 – A section through the vertebral column

- the *neural or vertebral arch* – a strong arch of bone enclosing the vertebral foramen. It is made up of several fused parts. It protects the spinal cord, which passes down from the brain through the vertebral foramen;
- the *spinous process* – a spikelike backward projection. It provides attachment for many muscles and ligaments;
- the *transverse process* – two projections, one on either side. They also provide attachment for muscles and ligaments;
- four *facets* – surfaces (two above and two below) for articulating with the adjacent vertebrae.

Spaces between the vertebrae known as the *inter-vertebral foramina* allow the passage of nerves entering and leaving the spinal cord along its length.

All vertebrae except the first and second cervical (atlas and axis) have these features in common, but they vary in size, becoming larger lower down for weight bearing. The fused vertebrae of the sacrum and coccyx also differ.

The inter-vertebral discs

These lie between the bodies of the vertebrae; they act as shock absorbers and allow for compression and distortion along the column. The core of the disc is the *nucleus pulposus*, which is a jelly-like material consisting of 85 per cent water. Surrounding this is the *annulus fibrosus*, which is composed of many rings of elastic fibres woven at angles to each other. It is thus able to expand and move to absorb compression forces.

As we grow older, the nucleus loses its water-binding capacity, fibro-cartilage replaces the gelatinous substance and the nucleus gradually hardens. The annulus fibrosus also loses its elasticity. As elasticity and flexibility are lost, the hardened rigid disc becomes more susceptible to injury. If the compression forces are abnormally strong or sudden, the annulus fibrosus may tear or rupture, allowing the nucleus to protrude into the space. This is known as a 'slipped disc' or disc prolapse. If this protrusion presses against a nerve as it passes out of the spinal canal through the inter-vertebral foramen, then neurological symptoms will be felt along the path of the nerve, for example if the prolapse is in the lumbar spine, pain, tingling, pins and needles, numbness may be felt down the leg.

Disc problems can occur at any time, but the likelihood increases as we get older. It is therefore extremely important to consider the age and medical condition of clients when giving any neck and trunk exercises. Failure to do so can result in very serious injury.

Movement of the spinal column

The vertebrae and discs are bound together by strong, powerful ligaments. There is very little movement between adjacent vertebrae, but the total combined movement along the whole length allows considerable movement of the trunk. The movements of the vertebral column are:

- flexion
- extension
- side flexion
- rotation

There is a greater range of movement in the cervical and lumbar regions than in the thoracic. These variations are due to the length and direction of the spinous processes, the ratio between the height of the discs and the height of the vertebral body, and the tension of the supporting ligaments.

Flexion and extension of the neck occur in the cervical region. Flexion and extension of the trunk occur mainly in the lumbar region. Rotation of the trunk occurs mainly in the thoracic region.

Dangerous movements

The most hazardous movement is trunk forward flexion, as this movement takes place mainly in the lumbar spine; the leverage is long being the length of the head and trunk. About 20 per cent of the movement occurs between the fourth and fifth lumbar vertebrae, and 60 to 70 per cent occurs between the fifth lumbar vertebra and the first sacral vertebra. There is therefore a high risk of damage to this vulnerable area of the lower back. Hyperextension is also hazardous due to the extreme compression forces on the discs which may rupture.

The curves of the vertebral column

The vertebral column shows curves along its length. These are seen in the cervical, thoracic, lumbar and sacral regions. The thoracic and sacral curves are primary curves, being present before birth. The cervical and lumbar curves are secondary curves and develop after birth. The cervical curve develops when the baby lifts its head, the lumbar curve develops as the baby learns to sit and stand. When viewed posteriorly:

- the cervical curve is concave;
- the thoracic curve is convex;
- the lumbar curve is concave;
- the sacral curve is convex.

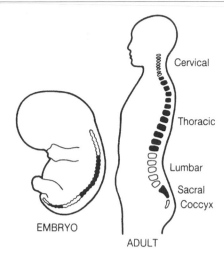

FIGURE NUMBER: 2.18 – Vertebral curves in the embryo and adult.

Spinal problems

Certain spinal problems result in exaggerated or abnormal spinal curves. When the spine is viewed posteriorly the following curves may be seen:

- *Kyphosis* is an exaggerated thoracic curve with increased convexity and forward flexion.
- *Lordosis* is an exaggerated lumbar curve with increased concavity and extension.
- *Kypho-lordosis* is a combination of the above.
- *Scoliosis* is a lateral deviation of the spine. It may deviate to the right or to the left and may show a long C curve or an S curve.

These curves are accompanied by muscle imbalance: some muscles will be too tight and the opposite groups will be over-stretched. Exercises can help to correct these problems.

These problems are fully discussed in Chapter 11.

TASKS

Work with a partner.

- Examine your partner's back and identify the five regions of the vertebral column.
- Run your index finger firmly down the spinous processes, leaving a red line. If the line deviates to the right or left it indicates a spinal problem. Name this spinal problem.
- Perform all the movements of the vertebral column.

The thorax or thoracic cavity

This is the bony cage of the chest, composed of the sternum, the 24 ribs and the twelve thoracic vertebrae.

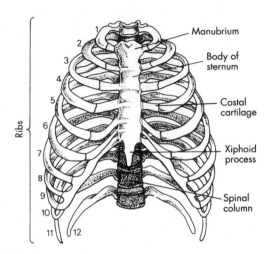

FIGURE NUMBER: 2.19 – Skeleton of the thorax.

The sternum

The sternum or breast bone is a flat narrow bone made up of three parts:

- the *manubrium* – the top part, squarish in shape;
- the *body* – the long middle part;
- the *xiphoid process* – the small pointed lower end.

The ribs

The ribs are narrow flat bones articulating with the thoracic vertebrae behind and with the sternum in front. The ribs are arranged in pairs, one on the right and the other on the left:

- Seven pairs are true ribs, which join the sternum.
- Five pairs are false ribs, which join the rib above. Two of these are called floating ribs as they have no attachment in front.

Each rib is joined to the sternum or to the adjacent ribs by a strip of hyaline cartilage. These are called the costal cartilages.

Small muscles known as the **intercostal muscles** fill the spaces between the ribs. They lie in two layers; eleven *internal intercostals* and eleven *external intercostals* on each side of the chest. a large muscle called the *diaphragm* forms the floor of the thoracic cavity. The lungs lie within and are protected by the thoracic cavity.

The mechanism of breathing

The capacity of the thorax must increase so that air can be taken in and then must decrease so that air can be forced out. During inspiration (breathing in), the intercostal muscles contract and swing the ribs upwards and outwards; the sternum is pushed forwards, and the diaphragm moves downwards. Thus the capacity of the thorax increases sideways, forwards and downwards and the pressure inside the thorax is lowered. When the pressure is reduced below atmospheric pressure (i.e. the pressure of the air outside the body), air rushes in and fills the lungs. Oxygen passes into the bloodstream through the walls of the capillaries surrounding the lungs and carbon dioxide passes the other way. During expiration (breathing out) the intercostal muscles relax, the diaphragm moves upwards, the ribs and sternum collapse back and the lungs recoil. This increases the pressure in the lungs and air is forced out.

During exercise, more oxygen is required to maintain energy for muscle contraction. Therefore the intercostals and diaphragm work harder and as a result they improve in strength and condition. The elasticity and condition of the lungs improves in the same way.

LEARN
During inspiration (breathing in) the following actions take place:
- Intercostals contract – ribs swing out and up
- Sternum pulled forward
- Diaphragm moves down

These actions increase the size of the chest cavity and air rushes in and fills the lungs.
- During expiration (breathing out):
- Intercostals relax
- Sternum moves back
- Diaphragm moves up
- Air is squeezed out as lungs recoil.

Air moves in and out of the lungs due to a difference in pressure. It moves from areas of high pressure to low pressure.

TASKS
- Place your hands on the sides of the lower ribs.
  Breathe in deeply and feel the ribs moving outwards and upwards. Breathe out and feel the ribs moving back.
  Repeat six times.
- Repeat this procedure with the hands over:
  a) the front of the midriff – breathe in and the abdomen moves out, breathe out:
  b) the body of the sternum – breathe in and the sternum swings forward, breathe out.

The girdles

There are two girdles, the pelvic girdle and the shoulder girdle.

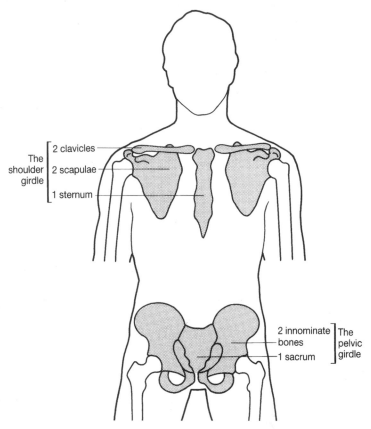

The
shoulder
girdle { 2 clavicles
2 scapulae
1 sternum

2 innominate
bones
1 sacrum } The
pelvic
girdle

FIGURE NUMBER: 2.20 – The shoulder and pelvic girdles.

> ### LEARN
> The pelvic girdle is made up of two innominate (pelvic bones) and the sacrum
> The shoulder girdle is made up of:
> ▪ two clavicles
> ▪ two scapulae

The pelvic girdle (or pelvis)

This is the circle of bone commonly called the hips. It protects various organs, for example the uterus and bladder, and transmits body weight to the legs. It is shaped rather like a basin and has an inner and outer surface.

The pelvic girdle is made up of three bones – two innominate bones and the sacrum (part of the vertebral column).

The two large innominate or pelvic bones articulate in front at a cartilaginous joint called the *pubic symphysis*. At the back they articulate on each side of the sacrum at gliding synovial joints called the *sacro-iliac joints*. There is hardly any movement at these joints as they fit tightly together and are held in place by very strong ligaments. The pelvis is supported on the femoral heads and may tilt forward, backward or sideways. Pelvic tilt accompanies movements of the trunk and hip joints, as is shown in chapter 4.

The shoulder girdle (the pectoral girdle)

The shoulder girdle is composed of two clavicles in front and two scapulae at the back. Anteriorly, each clavicle articulates with the sternum at the *sterno-clavicular joint*. Laterally, the clavicles articulate with the acromion process of the scapula at the *acromio-clavicular joint*.

The shoulder girdle forms an incomplete ring of bone around the upper thorax, joining the upper limbs to the axial skeleton.

The movement of the shoulder girdle accompany movements of the shoulder joint and contribute to a wide range of arm movements.

> **LEARN**
>
> The pelvic girdle is a rigid structure and contributes little to the movement of the hip joint and leg but the shoulder girdle is freely moveable and contributes greatly to the wide range of movement of the shoulder joint and arm.

Response to exercise

Bone tissue will adapt in response to exercise, and the degree of improvement relates to the intensity of the applied forces. Adaptation will occur only in those bones subjected to stress. The adaptations include:

- Increased enzyme activity which improves the condition of the bones
- Increased strength of bones reducing the risk of fractures
- Increase in bone girth following intense weight training programmes
- Increased bone mineral density: the deposits of minerals such as calcium increase in response to the stresses applied to the bones.

Exercise and increased calcium intake is particularly beneficial for post menopausal women as it can delay and protect against osteoporosis. This is condition where calcium is lost, bones become brittle and fracture easily.

Summary and aid to learning

The skeleton can be thought of in two parts; the axial and appendicular part:

- *The axial skeleton* is the central part. It includes: the skull, vertebral column, ribs, sternum and hyoid.
- *The appendicular skeleton* includes all the bones of the limbs, i.e the shoulder, arm, hand, hip, leg, foot.

■ List all the bones of the appendicular skeleton.

The vertebral column or spinal column is made up of separate bones called *vertebrae* (the singular is *vertebra*). In between the bodies of the vertebrae, are discs of fibro-cartilage, which act as shock absorbers; these are called *intervertebral* discs.

The medical term 'slipped disc' refers to movement or damage of one or more of these discs. The condition causes pain because the displaced disc may press on a nerve leaving the spinal cord. Spinal nerves leave the spinal cord through a small space found between the vertebrae, called the *intervertebral foramen*.

The vertebral column is divided into five regions: the cervical region, the thoracic region, the lumbar region, the sacrum and the coccyx; the bones of the sacrum and coccyx are fused together.

Read the text, list the regions of the vertebral column and give the number of vertebrae in each region.

Which region is most vulnerable to damage?

The major parts of a typical vertebra are: the body, neural arch, spinous process, two transverse processes and four facets.
Examine a vertebra and identify each part.

Work with a partner to perform the movements of the spinal column then identify each movement: discuss the movements which may cause damage and give reasons why they are hazardous. Think of exercises that you would avoid including in any exercise plan because they involve these movements.

The thorax is the chest area. It is made up of: the sternum in front, 12 pairs of ribs and the 12 thoracic vertebrae. The diaphragm, a large muscle, forms the base and separates the thoracic cavity from the abdominal cavity. In the spaces between the ribs lie the intercostal muscles. These muscles expand the chest during breathing.

Explain the difference between true ribs, false ribs and floating ribs. Examine a skeleton and point these out to a friend.

The shoulder girdle is an incomplete ring of bone around the top of the trunk. It is made up of the two clavicles and the sternum in front, and the two scapulae behind. It is a freely moveable structure.

The pelvic girdle is a complete ring of bone around the base of the trunk. It is made up of two innominate or pelvic bones and the sacrum. It is a very rigid structure.

Explain why the shoulder girdle contributes to the movement of the shoulder joint but the pelvic girdle does not contribute to the movement of the hip joint.

QUESTIONS

1. Compare the two main divisions of the human skeleton.
2. List the bones in each division.
3. Explain the functions of the skeletal system.
4. Explain why cancellous bone is sometimes known as spongy bone.
5. List the four main types of bones and give one example of each.
6. Describe the anatomical position.
7. Define the following terms:
   a anterior surface
   b proximal end
   c medial
   d superior structure
   e deep muscle
8. List the bones of the skull.
9. Name the regions of the vertebral column and give the number of vertebrae in each.
10. Give two functions of the inter-vertebral discs.
11. Compare the following spinal problems: kyphosis, lordosis, scoliosis.
12. List the bones that form the thoracic cavity or thorax.
13. Where is the xiphold process located?
14. Explain the terms true and false ribs.
15. Label the diagram below:

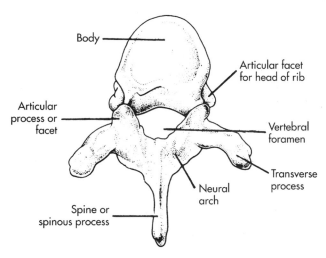

FIGURE NUMBER: 2.21 – A typical vertebra.

Chapter 3
The joints of the skeletal system

JOINTS

When two or more bones meet they form a joint, sometimes called an articulation. All body movement occurs at joints, from the small movements of the fingers to the large movements of the shoulder. The bones are held together by connective tissue and are moved by the contraction of skeletal muscle.

The shape of the articulating bones and the flexibility and tensile strength of the surrounding connective tissue determines the strength, stability and movement of joints.

Bones with curved surfaces that fit into each other and are close together form strong stable joints with less movement. Bones with little curvature that fit together loosely form joints that are less stable but allow greater movement.

> **LEARN**
> A joint is formed when two or more bones meet. It is sometimes referred to as an articulation.

THE TERMINOLOGY OF JOINT MOVEMENT

The following terms are used to describe the direction of joint movement:

- *flexion* – the bringing together of two surfaces (a bending movement), (e.g. bending the elbow or knee);
- *extension* – movement in the opposite direction to flexion (a straightening movement), (e.g. straightening the elbow or knee);
- *abduction* – movement away from the mid-line (e.g. taking the arm away from the body);
- *adduction* – movement towards the mid-line (e.g. taking the arm back to the body);
- *rotation* – movement around a long axis, which may be medial rotation (e.g. turning the arm in) or lateral rotation (e.g. turning the arm out);
- *circumduction* – a movement where the limb describes a cone whose apex lies in the joint: a combination of flexion, abduction, extension and adduction (e.g. circling the shoulder joint or hip joint round and round).

Movements that occur between the radius and ulna:
- *supination* turns the hand forwards or upwards;
- *pronation* turns the hand backwards or downwards.

Movements of the ankle joint:
- *dorsi-flexion* – pulling the foot upwards;
- *plantar flexion* – pointing the foot downwards.

Movements of the foot (occurring between the tarsal joints):
- *inversion* – turning the sole of the foot inwards;
- *eversion* – turning the sole of the foot outwards.

Movements of the shoulder girdle (and jaw):
- *elevation* – lifting the shoulder (jaw) upwards;
- *depression* – dropping the shoulders (jaw);
- *protraction* – drawing the shoulders (jaw) forward;
- *retraction* – drawing the shoulders (jaw) backwards.

Movements of the head and trunk:
- *forward flexion* – bending the head or trunk forward;
- *side flexion* – bending the head or trunk to the side. It may be right side flexion or left side flexion;
- *extension* – moving the head or trunk backwards;
- *rotation* – turning the head or trunk to the right or to the left, a twisting movement;
- *circumduction* – moving the head or trunk in a circular motion.

The terminology used to describe joint movement must be understood. Learning these thoroughly now makes muscle work much easier later on.

Some joints only move in two directions, for example the elbow and knee, whilst others will move in six directions, for example the shoulder and hip joints. As has previously been mentioned, muscles pull on the bones to produce these movements. Therefore some muscles will be *flexors*, producing flexion at the joint, whilst other muscles will be *extensors*, producing extension at the joint, and so on. When one group of muscles contracts to produce movement (the agonists) the opposite groups must relax to allow the movement to take place (the antagonists). See page 00.

THE CLASSIFICATION OF JOINTS

There are three main groups:

- *Fibrous* joints are immovable. The bones fit tightly together and are held firmly by fibrous tissue. There is no joint cavity. Examples are the sutures of the skull.
- *Cartilaginous* joints are slightly movable. The bones are connected by a disc of fibro-cartilage. There is no joint cavity. Examples are the symphysis pubis (between the pubic bones) and the inter-vertebral joints (between the vertebral bodies).
- *Synovial* joints are freely movable. These are the most numerous in the body. There are six different types of synovial joints. They are classified according to their planes of movement, which depend on the shape of the articulating bones. All the freely movable joints of the body are synovial joints and although their shape and movements vary, they all have certain characteristics in common.

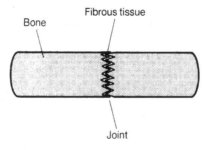

FIGURE NUMBER: 3.1 – A fibrous joint.

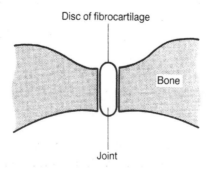

FIGURE NUMBER: 3.2 – A cartilaginous joint.

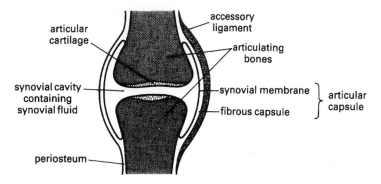

FIGURE NUMBER: 3.3 – A synovial joint.

> *LEARN*
>
> There are three main types of joints:
> - Fibrous – no movement
> - Cartilaginous – slight movement
> - Synovial – freely moveable

Features of a typical synovial joint

- A joint cavity (space within the joint)
- Hyaline cartilage, which covers the surfaces of the articulating bones. Sometimes called articular cartilage, it reduces friction and allows smooth movement. As previously mentioned, with age, injury or disease there may be erosion or damage of this cartilage. Friction will increase as bone moves over bone, the joint will be stiff and movements painful. Regular exercise will delay the onset of these problems, but if there is joint damage exercises must only be performed under medical supervision
- The capsule or articulating capsule, which surrounds the joint like a sleeve. It holds the bones together and encloses the cavity. The capsule is strengthened on the outside by ligaments, which help to stabilise and strengthen the joints. Ligaments may also be found inside a joint, holding the bones together in order to increase stability. The movement at any joint will be limited by the tightness or rigidity of the capsule and ligaments. Flexibility exercises and full-range mobility exercises will maintain and increase the extensibility of these structures and maintain full-range joint movement
- The synovial membrane lining the capsule, which produces synovial fluid
- Synovial fluid or synovium, a viscous fluid which lubricates and nourishes the joint. Regular exercise stimulates an increase in the production of synovial fluid, so that lubrication and nourishment of the cartilage is increased.

Discs (menisci)

Some joints, such as the knee, have pads of fibro-cartilage called discs. They are attached to the bones and give the joint a better 'fit'. They also cushion movement. These structures are prone to damage and tearing, usually as a result of excessive stress and rotational forces.

Classification of the six synovial joints

Table 3.1 The synovial joints		
Type of joint	Examples	Movements
Gliding joints	intercarpal and intertarsal joints	multiaxial; movements limited to gliding or shifting
Hinge joints	elbow, knee, ankle, interphalangeal joints (joints of fingers and toes)	uniaxial and one plane only (sagittal plane, frontal axis); movements – flexion and extension
Pivot joints	superior radio-ulnar joint and atlas on axis (moves the head left and right)	uniaxial and one plane only (horizontal plane, vertical axis); movement – rotation
Ellipsoid (condyloid) joints	wrist (radio-carpal), knuckle (metacarpo phalangeal joint)	biaxial and in two planes (frontal and sagittal axes, sagittal and frontal planes); movements – flexion, extension, adduction, abduction, circumduction
Saddle joints	carpo-metacarpal joint of thumb (base of thumb)	multiaxial – sagittal, frontal and vertical axes with corresponding planes; movements – flexion, extension, adduction, abduction, rotation (limited), circumduction
Ball and socket joints	hip and shoulder joints	multiaxial – sagittal, frontal and vertical axes with corresponding planes; movements – flexion, extension, adduction, abduction, rotation (medial and lateral), circumduction

LEARN

Parts of a synovial joint are:

- Joint cavity
- Hyaline cartilage – covers bone ends
- Capsule surrounds the joint like a sleeve, ligaments around the joint strengthen the capsule
- Synovial membrane – lines capsule and secretes synovial fluid
- Synovial fluid lubricates the joint and nourishes the cartilage

Bursae

Any movement produces friction between the moving parts. In order to reduce friction, sac-like structures containing synovial fluid are found between tissues. These are called *bursae* and are usually found between tendons and bone. They may become inflamed following injury or repetitive stress. This results in swelling, stiffness and pain of the joint.

> **LEARN**
>
> Ligaments are found outside and sometimes inside the joint. They are tough bands of connective tissue which help to hold the bones together.

> **LEARN**
>
> The range or degree of movement at a joint will depend on:
> - The shape of the articulating surfaces of the bones
> - The tension of the capsule and ligaments
> - The tension of muscles and tendons around the joint
> - The contact between the soft tissue around the joint
> - Age

THE RANGE OF MOVEMENT AT JOINTS

The range and degree of movement at joints will vary from individual to individual and will depend on many factors. An understanding of these factors will enable the therapist to plan realistic objectives and avoid being over-ambitious.

- *The shape and contour of the articulating surfaces.* The range of movement will be limited when the bones fit tightly into each other. Examine the hip and shoulder joints: both are synovial ball and socket joints capable of the same number of movements, but the shoulder joint allows a far greater range than the hip joint. This is because the shoulder has a shallow socket (the glenoid cavity) for articulating with the large ball (the head of the humerus) so the movement is not restricted by the depth of the socket. The hip, on the other hand, has a deep socket (acetabulum) into which the head of the femur fits tightly and securely restricting movement.
- *The tension of the connective tissue components* – the capsule and the ligaments supporting the joint. Ligaments are made of tough, non-elastic, white fibrous tissue. They are found strengthening the capsule around the outside of joints and sometimes inside the joints. They hold the bones together to stabilise and support the joint. They are particularly important for loosely-fitting joints such as the shoulder and weight-bearing joints such as the knee. These ligaments prevent abnormal movements, but if a joint is pushed beyond its range with great enough force these ligaments may tear. Ligaments

may be partially torn, as in sprains, or they may rupture completely and the joint may dislocate.

- *The tension of muscles and tendons around the joint*. Tight muscles will limit the movement in underlying joints. Cold muscles are not as extensible as warm muscles and their tension may prevent full joint movement. Forcing a joint when the muscles around it are cold may result in tears or strains of the muscle fibres. It is therefore important to perform warm-up routines before exercising joints through their full range. Some muscles, such as the hamstrings, pass over two joints and the position of one joint limits movement in the other. Note the difference in the range of movement when flexing the hip with the knee straight and flexing the hip with the knee bent. The range of movement is far greater in the latter.

- *The approximation of soft tissue near the joint*. Joint movement is limited when surfaces come into contact with each other, preventing further movement, for example, flexion of the elbow joint is limited when the muscles of the forearm touch the biceps.

- *Ageing* will affect joint range. Children are more supple than young adults, and the young adults more supple than the elderly, because tissues and ligaments tighten with age. Good regular exercise routines will help to maintain range. So called double-jointed people have a greater range of joint movement because they are born with lax ligaments.

Because of the importance of joint movements in exercises, the basic structure and movements of each joint must be clearly understood. This knowledge enables the therapist to select appropriate exercises to maintain range and mobility and, most importantly, to give advice on the prevention of injury, i.e. strains, sprains, dislocation and fractures.

THE MAJOR FEATURES OF SKELETAL JOINTS

TASKS
- Examine diagrams 3.4–3.11 and learn the major features.
- Examine models of joints and identify the major features.
- Relate each joint to your own body and perform the possible movement.
- Working in pairs, ask your partner to perform named movements, such as flexion of the hip joint or extension of the knee joint.

JOINTS OF THE LEG (LOWER LIMB)

The hip joint
Type: Synovial – ball and socket
Bones: The head of the femur articulates with the acetabulum of the innominate bone

Movements: Flexion, extension (sagittal plane)
Abduction, adduction (frontal plane)
Rotation (medial and lateral) (horizontal plane)
Circumduction (a combination of flexion
abduction, extension and adduction).

True flexion and extension of the hip joint are limited to 90° flexion and only 10° extension, but these movements are greatly increased by tilting and rotation of the pelvis forwards and backwards and by associated movements of the vertebral column.

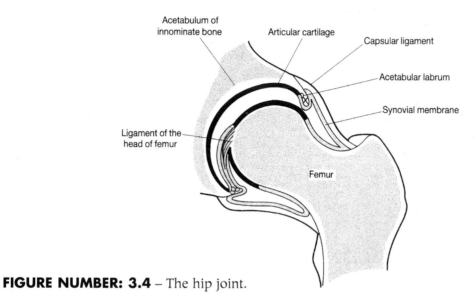

FIGURE NUMBER: 3.4 – The hip joint.

The knee joint

Type: Synovial – hinge
Bones: The condyles of the femur articulate with the condyles of the tibia. (The posterior aspect of the patella also articulates)
Movements: Flexion and extension (sagittal plane). In flexion there is slight rotation

The knee joint is susceptible to many injuries as its stability depends on its powerful ligaments and muscles. Severe stresses can cause sprains, tears or ruptures of any of the ligaments, i.e. the medial and lateral collateral ligaments or the cruciate ligaments. The menisci or cartilages may also be damaged and may require surgical removal.

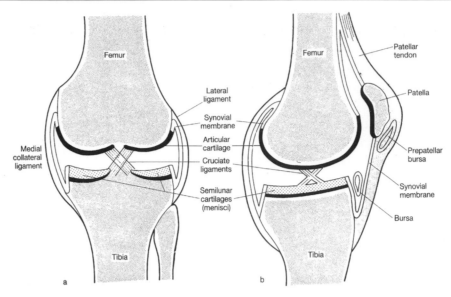

FIGURE NUMBER: 3.5 – The knee joint. (a) Viewed from the front. (b) Viewed from the side.

The ankle joint

Type: Synovial – hinge
Bones: The malleoli of the tibia and fibula articulate with the talus
Movements: Plantar flexion – pointing toe down (flexion)
               Dorsi-flexion – pulling foot up (extension)

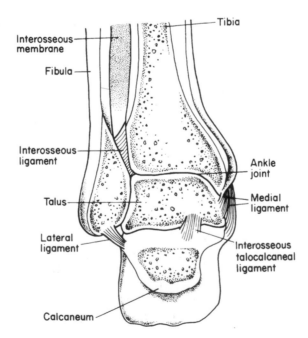

FIGURE NUMBER: 3.6 – The ankle joint.

The subtalar and talo-calcaneo navicular joints

Type: Synovial – gliding
Bones: Tarsal bones
Movements: Inversion – turning sole inwards
                Eversion – turning sole outwards

The ligaments around the ankle joint are susceptible to injury, a condition commonly called sprained ankle. The lateral ligament is the most vulnerable as there is a greater range of inversion if the ankle is forced inward. However, tears of the medial ligament occur in forced eversion injuries. Forced plantar flexion will tear the capsular ligament anteriorly.

The joints of the foot

The 26 bones of the foot articulate with each other, forming a variety of joints. The bones of the foot form three arches, which help to absorb shock and prevent jarring during walking, running, etc.

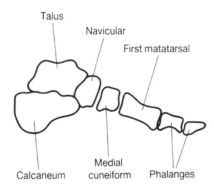

FIGURE NUMBER: 3.7 – The Medial arch of the foot.

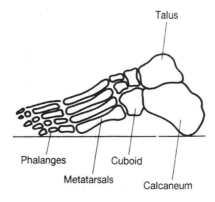

FIGURE NUMBER: 3.8 – The lateral arch of the foot.

■ The *medial arch* runs along the inside of the foot from the heel (calcaneus) to the three medial toes. This arch is supported by the tendons of the tibialis anterior and tibialis posterior muscles, which act as slings lifting the arch. Normally this arch is not in contact with the ground during weight bearing. If the muscles and ligaments are weak, the arch drops to create the condition known as flat feet. If the muscles and ligaments are tight the arch is held high, and this is known as high instep.

■ The *lateral arch* runs along the outside of the foot from the heel to the two lateral toes. This arch is supported by the tendons of the peroneus longus and peroneus brevis muscles. This is low to the ground and transmits body weight from the heel along the outer border of the foot to the toes during weight bearing.

■ The *anterior transverse arch* lies under the ball of the foot along the metatarsal heads. It is supported by ligaments and the lumbrical muscles. Collapse of this arch can lead to severe pain under the metatarsal heads. Numerous ligaments and small muscles support these bones in the sole of the foot. They are arranged in four layers, and are protected and separated from the skin by the plantar fascia.

Two important ligaments are:
■ the spring ligament, which passes from calcaneus to navicular;
■ the long plantar ligament, which passes from calcaneus to cuboid and the middle three metatarsals.

The movements of the foot during walking and running are very complex and good foot function is essential to prevent stresses in higher joints. The walking action should begin by striking with the heel, then transfer the weight to the outer border and push off from the toes. The skin over the sole, meanwhile, relays important sensory stimuli to the brain. Impaired foot function can give rise to many problems, such as poor co-ordination, strains on ligaments, stresses at joints and impairment of the function of muscles, with accompanying pain and stiffness. Care of the feet is a priority for everyone partaking in sport and exercise, and choice of footwear is exceedingly important.

JOINTS OF THE ARM (UPPER LIMB)

The shoulder

Type: Synovial – ball and socket
Bones: The head of the humerus articulates with the glenoid cavity of the scapula
Movement: Flexion and extension, abduction and adduction, rotation (medial and lateral), circumduction

The range of movement at the shoulder joint is greatly increased by accompanying movements of the shoulder girdle.

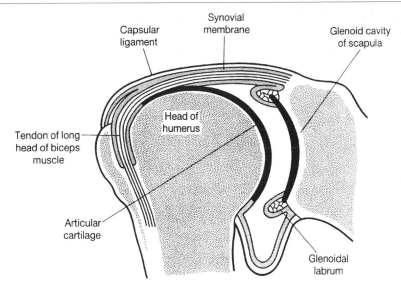

FIGURE NUMBER: 3.9 – The shoulder joint.

The elbow joint

Type: Synovial – hinge joint

Bones: The trochlea of the humerus articulates with the trochlear notch of the ulna and the head of the radius with the capitulum of the humerus

Movements: Flexion and extension

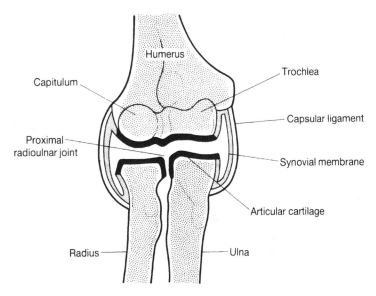

FIGURE NUMBER: 3.10 – The elbow joint.

The superior radio-ulnar joint
Type: Synovial – pivot
Bones: The head of the radius articulates with the radial notch of the ulna
Movements: Pronation and supination

The wrist joint
Type: Synovial – ellipsoid (condyloid)
Bones: The lower end of the radius and disc of the ulna articulate with the scaphoid, lunate and triquetral
Movements: Flexion and extension, abduction and adduction, circumduction

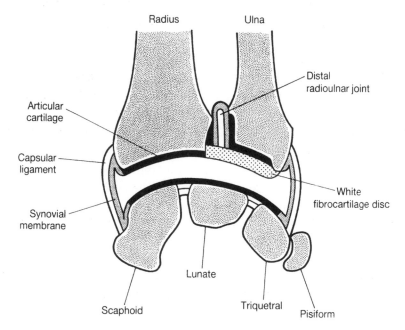

FIGURE NUMBER: 3.11 – The wrist joint.

Response to exercise
Ligaments and tendons increase in strength in response to training and their flexibility also increases. These connective tissue components are therefore more able to accommodate any increased or excessive forces applied to them. This improvement in tensile strength reduces the risk of injury.

Joint function improves as there is an increase in synovial fluid to the joint which lubricates the joint, facilitating movement.

The cartilage is nourished and lubricated which improves its condition and the function of the joint.

Following a programme of training there is an increase in the thickness of the hyaline cartilage which increases its cushioning properties.

Summary and aid to learning

A joint is formed when two or more bones meet.

All body movement takes place at joints. Muscles produce the movement by contracting and pulling on bones, then the movement takes place at the joint.

Some joints allow more movement than others; this is largely dependent on the shape of the articulating surfaces.

Read the text and learn all the terminology regarding movement. Then, with a partner, consider every joint and work out every movement possible at each joint.

There are three main groups of joints:
- *Fibrous joints* – held together with fibrous tissue and are immovable.
- *Cartilaginous joints* – have a disc of cartilage between the bones. There is a slight amount of shifting movement at these joints.
- *Synovial joints* – contain synovial fluid secreted by the synovial membrane, which lubricates the joint. These joints are freely moveable.

Can you give an example of each of the joints listed above?

There are six different types of synovial joint. Name these joints and give one example of each.

Draw an example of a typical synovial joint and label the following parts: joint cavity, synovial membrane, hyaline cartilage, capsule, ligaments and synovial fluid.

QUESTIONS

1. Define the term articulation.
2. List the three main groups of joints and give an example from each group.
3. Give the functions of the following parts of a synovial joint:
   a the synovial membrane
   b the synovial fluid
   c the hyaline cartilage.
4. Name one joint where discs or menisci are to be found.
5. List the six types of synovial joint.
6. Briefly explain any four factors that limit the range of movement at joints.
7. List and define the movements of the hip joint.
8. Give two reasons why there is a greater range of movement in the shoulder joint compared with the hip joint, although both are ball and socket.
9. Give the movements of the ankle joint (remember that this is a hinge joint).
10. Name and describe the arches of the foot.
11. Describe the action of walking.
12. Name and describe the movements that occur between the radius and ulna.
13. Explain briefly how bones, ligaments and tendons improve in response to exercise.

Chapter 4
Skeletal muscle

Skeletal muscle forms the body flesh and gives the body shape. It is able to generate great force to produce and control movement. It possesses *three* important properties:

- ■ *Contractability* – this is the ability to contract and shorten in response to a stimulus from the central nervous system.
- ■ *Extensibility* – this is the ability to lengthen while generating force or contracting, if it is acted on by an external force.
- ■ *Elasticity* – this is the ability to return to its relaxed normal length after it has been stretched, rather like a piece of elastic.

Muscle tissue is totally under the control of the nervous system. Muscles are richly supplied with blood vessels and nerves, both sensory and motor. Stimuli initiated in the brain are transmitted via motor nerves to the muscle fibres resulting in their contraction. As large numbers of muscle fibres are stimulated to contract, the whole muscle contracts and shortens. This shortening of the muscle exerts a force on the bones of attachment resulting in movement.

In addition to producing movement, muscle tissue has other important functions.

Functions of skeletal muscle tissue

Producing movement – as explained above, this is the main function of skeletal muscle. When muscles are stimulated to contract, they exert a force or pull on bones at their point of attachment which results in movement at the joint.

Maintaining posture – muscles maintain the upright posture. A proportion of fibres within a muscle will contract to keep the body upright.

Generating heat – the metabolic processes involved in energy release during muscle contraction produces heat, the harder and longer the contraction the greater the heat produced. The body uses muscle contraction to produce heat if the body temperature falls too low. We are all familiar with the process of shivering when we are cold and the body temperature falls below a certain level. Shivering is really small involuntary muscle contractions which produce heat and raise body temperature.

Stabilising joints – the muscles around a joint will help to support and stabilise the joint. While the prime mover is contracting to produce the required movement, other muscles will contract to stabilise the joint so that the prime mover can contract with maximum efficiency.

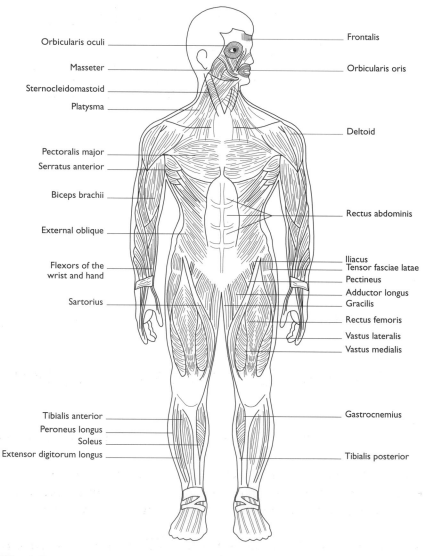

Orbicularis oculi
Masseter
Sternocleidomastoid
Platysma
Pectoralis major
Serratus anterior
Biceps brachii
External oblique
Flexors of the wrist and hand
Sartorius
Tibialis anterior
Peroneus longus
Soleus
Extensor digitorum longus

Frontalis
Orbicularis oris
Deltoid
Rectus abdominis
Iliacus
Tensor fasciae latae
Pectineus
Adductor longus
Gracilis
Rectus femoris
Vastus lateralis
Vastus medialis
Gastrocnemius
Tibialis posterior

FIGURE NUMBER: 4.1a – Anterior aspect showing body muscles.

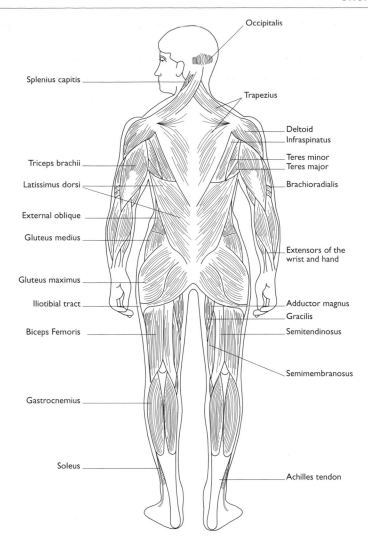

Occipitalis

Splenius capitis

Trapezius

Deltoid
Infraspinatus

Triceps brachii

Teres minor
Teres major

Latissimus dorsi

Brachioradialis

External oblique

Gluteus medius

Extensors of the
wrist and hand

Gluteus maximus

Iliotibial tract

Adductor magnus
Gracilis

Biceps Femoris

Semitendinosus

Semimembranosus

Gastrocnemius

Soleus

Achilles tendon

FIGURE NUMBER: 4.1b – Posterior aspect showing body muscles.

THE STRUCTURE OF SKELETAL MUSCLE

Skeletal muscle is composed of muscle fibres arranged in bundles called fasciculi; many bundles of fibres make up the complete muscle. The fibres, bundles and muscles are surrounded and protected by connective tissue sheaths:

- The connective tissue around each fibre is called the *endomysium*.
- The connective tissue around each bundle is called the *perimysium*.
- The connective tissue around the muscle is called the *epimysium*.

This connective tissue blends at each end of the muscle to form tendons which attach the muscles to the underlying bones.

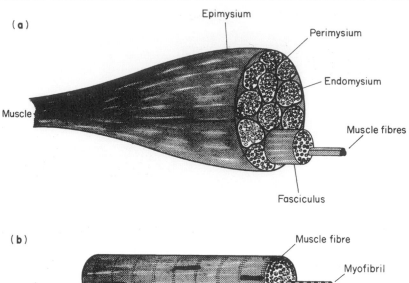

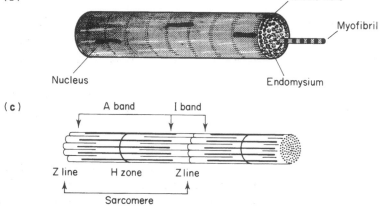

FIGURE NUMBER: 4.2 – (a) The structure of a muscle.
(b) A single muscle fibre showing striations.
(c) A myofibril, illustrating a sarcomere.

LEARN
Muscles are composed of:
- Muscle fibres covered by the endomysium (lots of fibres together form bundles)
- Muscle bundles covered by the perimysium (lots of bundles form the muscle)

The muscle is covered by the epimysium

Muscle fibres

Muscle fibres are long, thin multi-nucleate cells. The fibres vary from 10 to 100 microns in diameter and from a few millimetres to many centimetres in length. The long fibres extend the full length of the muscle, while the short fibres end in connective tissue intersections within the muscle.

Each muscle fibre is bound by a cell membrane known as the *sarcolemma*, just beneath which lie the nuclei. The cytoplasm of the muscle cell is known as the *sarcoplasm*. It contains large

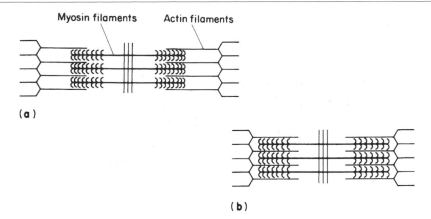

Myosin filaments   Actin filaments

(a)

(b)

FIGURE NUMBER: 4.3 – The sarcomere. (a) During relaxation. (b) During contraction.

numbers of mitochondria and other organelles. Muscle fibres are made up of smaller protein threads called *myofibrils*. These run the whole length of the fibre and are the elements which contract and relax. Myofibrils are made up of even smaller threads called *myofilaments*.

Under an electron microscope, myofibrils are seen to have alternate light and dark bands called I and A bands. In the middle of the dark A band is a lighter zone, the H zone. In the middle of the light I band is a dark line, the Z line.

The segment between two Z lines is known as the *sarcomere*. These sarcomeres are repeated along the whole length of the myofibril. Each sarcomere contains overlapping thick and thin myofilaments. The thin myofilaments are made of the protein *actin*. They begin at the Z line and extend into the A band, where they overlap with the thick myofilaments, which are made of the protein *myosin*. These thick bands have small cross-bridges projecting sideways towards active sites on the thin bands. These are very important: when a stimulus from the nervous system is received by the muscle fibre, a series of chemical reactions takes place which results in the cross-bridges linking and pulling the thin bands towards the thick bands. The sliding thin bands pull on the Z lines and each sarcomere shortens. Consequently, the myofibrils and fibres shorten and the whole muscle contracts. The energy for this contraction is obtained from the breakdown of ATP (adenosine triphosphate) stored in the myosine cross-bridges.

Muscle relaxation occurs when no stimulus is received from the nervous system. The thin bands slide back to their precontracted state and the muscle relaxes.

Muscle elongation occurs only as a result of some pulling force on the muscle. This force may be the pull of antagonistic muscles (i.e. on the opposite side of the joint), the pull of gravity, the pull of weights, springs, etc., or manual pulling by oneself or another person. The fibres elongate because the thin filaments move away from the thick filaments and each sarcomere gets longer. The pull must allow at least one cross-bridge to remain intact; otherwise, the sarcomere will rupture. Strong forces can cause small tears within a muscle because the cross-bridges are no longer intact. During exercise and sports, excessive stress may result in muscle tears.

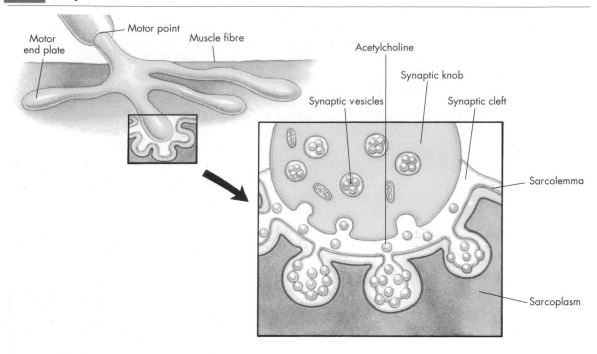

FIGURE NUMBER: 4.4 – Synapse.

Neuromuscular function

The contraction of skeletal muscle is controlled by the nervous system. When the brain receives information that movement is required, stimuli/impulses are initiated in the motor cortex which will activate the muscles to contract. These impulses, transmitted via motor nerve neurones, pass down from the brain via the spinal cord to the anterior horn cells. The axons of many anterior horn cells emerge together as a motor nerve and pass to a muscle.

The point at which the motor nerve enters the muscle is known as the *motor point*. Each axon will then divide into many branches and each branch will supply one muscle fibre.

The neuromuscular junction, i.e. the point at which the axon branch meets the muscle fibre, is known as the *motor end plate*.

The anterior horn cell, its axon, axon branches and all the muscle fibres it supplies, is known as a *motor unit*.

A stimulus of sufficient strength will result in all the muscle fibres within a motor unit contracting together to maximum strength but a stimulus below this intensity will not produce any response. The stimulus of sufficient intensity to produce a contraction is known as the *threshold stimulus*.

Remember that muscle fibres contract according to the 'all or none law' which states that **muscle fibres contract with maximum force or not at all**.

The number of motor units recruited will influence the strength of the contraction; the more motor units activated the greater the strength of the contraction. Strength training results in the recruitment of more motor units and hence greater muscle strength.

Another important consideration is the frequency of the impulses. A low frequency will produce a 'twitch' of the muscle, which is a quick contraction followed by complete relaxation. Increasing the frequency will result in a second contraction occurring before complete relaxation. The length of contraction will now be the sum of the two twitches; this will give a longer contraction and is known as *wave summation*. However, the contraction will not be smooth as the muscle will partially relax between the twitches. Increasing the frequency until the muscle cannot relax between stimuli will result in a smooth contraction of the muscle known as a *tetanic contraction*.

> *LEARN*
> The all or none law.
> When muscle fibres respond to a stimulus, they contract with maximum force or not at all.

Muscle fibre types

A muscle is composed of different types of muscle fibres which differ in their metabolism and function. The proportion of each fibre within a muscle will depend on the function of the muscle. There are two main types:

Type I   Red fibres:
Type II   White fibres: (which can be subdivided into type IIa, IIb and IIc).

Type I fibres are slow twitch fibres which are equipped to contract slowly but repeatedly over a long period of time and utilise the aerobic energy system. They are used during endurance activities such as marathon running or swimming.

Type II fibres are fast twitch fibres that are equipped to contract rapidly for short periods only and utilise the anaerobic energy systems. They are used in fast rapid activities such as squash or short sprints.

The different properties of the fibres are shown opposite.

Muscle shape

Muscle shape varies depending on the function of the muscle. The fleshy bulk of the muscle is known as the belly. The bundles of muscle fibres lie either parallel or obliquely to the line of pull of the muscle. Parallel fibres are found in strap-like and fusiform muscles. These long fibres allow

Type 1 Slow twitch	Type II Fast twitch
Utilises aerobic pathway	Utilises anaerobic pathway
High endurance capacity	Low endurance capacity
Slow contraction	Fast contraction
High resistance to fatigue	Low resistance to fatigue
Small fibre diameter	Large fibre diameter
Low phosphocreatine stores	High phosphocreatine stores
High capillary density	Low capillary density
Low glycogen stores	High glycogen stores
Low glycolytic enzyme stores	High glycolytic enzyme stores
High triglyceride stores	Low triglyceride stores
High myoglobin content	Medium myoglobin content

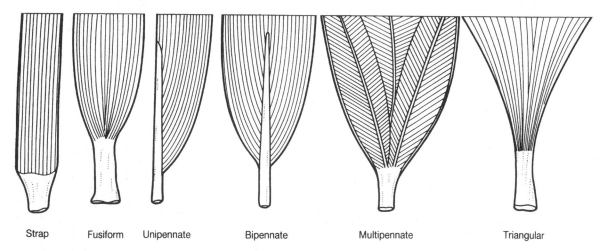

Strap   Fusiform   Unipennate   Bipennate   Multipennate   Triangular

FIGURE NUMBER: 4.5 – Muscle shape.

for a wide range of movement. The shorter oblique fibres are found in triangular and pennate muscles, where muscle strength is required.

Muscle attachments

As previously explained, a muscle is composed of muscle fibres and connective tissue components, namely the endomysium, perimysium and epimysium. Certain muscles have connective tissue intersections, dividing the muscle into several bellies, as seen in the rectus abdominus.

Sheets of connective tissue blend at either end of the muscle and attach the muscle to the underlying bones. Muscles are attached by either tendons or aponeuroses to the periosteum, the connective tissue covering the bone.

- *Tendons* are tough cord-like structures of connective tissue which attach muscles to bones.
- *Aponeuroses* are flat sheets of connective tissue which attach muscles along the length of the bone.

A muscle has at least two points of attachment, known as the *origin* and *insertion* of the muscle. These are attached on either side of the joint.

- The origin is usually proximal and stationary or immovable.
- The insertion is usually distal and movable.

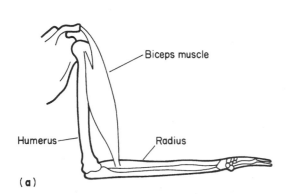
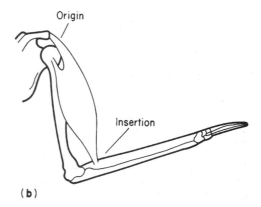

FIGURE NUMBER: 4.6 – The origin and insertion of a muscle.

> **LEARN**
> Muscles attach to bones by tendons or aponeuroses.
> There are at least two points where they attach called:
> - *Origin* – usually proximal and stationary
> - *Insertion* – usually distal and movable.

When muscles contract, it is usual for the insertion to move towards the origin, which remains stationary; however, certain muscles can also work in reverse, the origin moving towards the insertion. This is known as 'the reverse action of muscles' or 'origin-insertion reversed'. For example, the gluteus maximus extends the hip joint. When it pulls the leg backwards, the insertion on the femur moves towards the origin on the pelvis, which remains stationary. However, if the trunk is in forward flexion, the gluteus maximus can pull the trunk upright: then its origin on the pelvis moves towards the insertion on the femur, which remains stationary (see Figure 4.7).

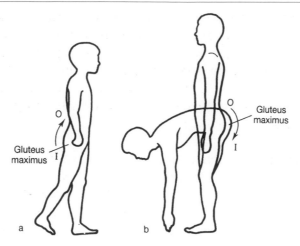

FIGURE NUMBER: 4.7 – Actions of gluteus maximus.

        (a) Extension of the hip joint, the insertion moves towards the origin.

        (b) Raising the trunk, the origin moves towards the insertion.

Muscle tone

Muscle tone is the state of partial contraction or tension found in muscles even when at rest. A small number of muscle fibres will always be in a state of contraction. The degree of tension will depend on the number of motor units recruited. The recruitment of a few motor units will be just sufficient to produce tautness in the muscle, but not to result in full contraction and movement. As different motor units are stimulated different groups of fibres will contract alternately, working a 'shift' system to prevent fatigue of the few. Changes in muscle tone are adjusted according to the information received from sensory receptors within the muscles and their tendons. *Muscle spindles* transmit information on the degree of stretch within the muscle. *Tendon receptors* called Golgi organs transmit information on the amount of tension applied to the tendon by muscle contraction. Too much stretch and tension will be counteracted by the recruitment of fewer motor units and a reduction in muscle tone. Too little will be counteracted by an increase in number of motor units and in muscle tone. Muscle tone is essential for maintaining upright posture.

- Hypotonic muscles, i.e. those with less than the normal degree of tone, are said to be flaccid.
- Hypertonic muscles, i.e. those with a greater degree of muscle tone and where fibres are over-contracted and rigid, are said to be spastic.
- A contraction that increases muscle tone but does not change the length of the muscle is called isometric contraction (equal length).
- A contraction where muscle tone remains the same but the muscle changes in length is called isotonic contraction (equal tone).

Blood supply to skeletal muscle

The oxygen and nutrients required by the contracting muscles are delivered by the circulating blood while the waste products of the energy-producing reactions are removed. During exercise there is a marked increase in blood flow to the exercising muscles. Blood is redirected from other organs such as the stomach and liver. Blood flow may increase from around 20 percent of cardiac output to 80 percent. The redirecting of blood from other areas is known as *blood shunting* or accommodation. The supplies of oxygen and nutrients are brought by the blood via the arteries, and the waste products are removed via the veins. The arteries branch to form smaller arteries and arterioles within the perimysium. They then divide further to form capillary networks within the endomysium, where they join venules, which lead to veins. When muscles are relaxed, the capillary network delivers blood to the muscle fibres.

When muscles contract, the pressure impedes the flow of blood through the capillary beds. This reduces the supply of oxygen and nutrients and limits the removal of waste. During exercise, muscle fibres alternately contract and relax and the capillaries deliver blood during the relaxation phase. However, repeated or sustained contraction, such as isometric work or exercising without sufficient rest periods, prevents the flow of blood to the muscle fibres, due to compression on the blood vessels and the capillaries. This results in muscle fatigue due to lack of oxygen and nutrients and the accumulation of waste products such as lactic acid. The strength and speed of contraction become progressively weaker, and as fatigue continues the muscle fails to relax completely, resulting in muscle spasm and pain. Regardless of the activity, muscles must be given sufficient time to relax completely. This will ensure an adequate blood supply and prevent fatigue.

Regular endurance aerobic exercise results in an increase in blood vessels and capillary networks to the muscles. This will improve the blood supply, increase levels of oxygen and nutrients and reduce levels of lactic acid. Thus the capacity to exercise without fatigue will improve.

Energy for muscle contraction

Energy may be defined as the ability or capacity to perform work. All human activity is dependent upon the ability to provide energy on a continuous basis, all tissue cells require energy to carry out their activities. Energy is provided by the food we eat but the energy liberated from the breakdown of food is not directly employed to do work but rather, is used to manufacture a chemical compound, adenosine triphosphate (ATP). The energy supplied by the breakdown of this high energy chemical compound provides the energy for cells to perform their work.

Muscle cells expend far more energy than other cells, and convert chemical energy to mechanical energy. Only a limited quantity of ATP is stored in muscle cells and this is depleted after a few seconds of activity and must be continually replenished if muscle contraction is to continue. The body has adapted different systems for the resynthesis of ATP and hence energy production. ATP may be resynthesised through the breakdown of another high energy chemical compound, namely phosphocreatine (PC), also stored in muscle cells, but the main source of energy is provided by carbohydrates and fats stored as glycogen in muscle cells and in the liver. If the energy is generated by reactions which do not utilise oxygen, they are *anaerobic* energy systems. If the reactions utilise oxygen, they are *aerobic* energy systems.

The system used will depend on the *intensity* and *duration* of the activity and on *the availability and use of oxygen.*

Remember that throughout the following text **ATP** represents adenosine triphosphate. **PC** represents phosphocreatine.

There are *three* energy systems for resynthesising ATP; two are anaerobic energy systems and one is the aerobic energy system.

The systems are:
- the **alactic** ATP – PC system or phosphagen system (anaerobic).
- the **lactic** acid system (anaerobic glycolysis).
- the **aerobic** (oxygen) system (aerobic glycolysis).

The alactic ATP – PC system

This system provides the most rapidly available source of energy as it utilises the ATP and PC stored in muscle cells. It does not depend on transporting oxygen from the lungs nor on a long chain of chemical reactions. Therefore when a muscle is stimulated to contract, immediate energy is obtained from stored ATP and the activity will continue for 5–6 seconds until the ATP is depleted. ATP is then replenished by the breakdown of PC. This supply will provide energy for 10–15 seconds of maximum effort, until the stored PC is depleted. This fast system would be used in activities of short duration such as sprinting, kicking, jumping, throwing actions and in the initial effort of push off from the starting block. The amount of energy obtainable from this system is limited due to the limited stores of ATP and PC in the muscle. However, they are replenished very quickly after three to four minutes of recovery. This is important as the rapid activity can be performed again after a short rest.

Oxygen is not utilised, therefore it is anaerobic.

The lactic acid system

If the activity continues after the stored phosphocreatine is depleted, ATP is resynthesised from glycogen (carbohydrate).

Carbohydrate is eaten as sugars and starch and converted to glycogen which is found in the blood and stored in muscle tissue and in the liver.

The breakdown of the glucose molecule to resynthesise ATP and hence provide energy, involves a series of reactions known as *glycolysis*. Initially, if oxygen is not available quickly enough, energy is liberated through the partial breakdown of glycogen known as *anaerobic glycolysis* which occurs in the intracellular fluid of the muscle cell.

The glycogen molecule is broken down to pyruvic acid which in the absence of oxygen is converted to lactic acid. This system utilises carbohydrate only.

This system is not particularly efficient as it yields only 2–3 moles of ATP for each molecule of glucose, which releases only a small amount of energy. However, it is an important source of fast energy for 2–3 minutes of high intensity activity such as 400–800 metre running or 100–200 metre swimming. It is also used at the end of a run during the final 'burst'.

Anaerobic glycolysis results in the formation of lactic acid which contributes to muscle fatigue. With the build of lactic acid within the muscle, contraction will diminish and activity will stop.

The aerobic system

This system of energy release requires a continuing supply of oxygen and is therefore termed the aerobic system. When oxygen is available, glycogen is completely broken down through a series of complicated reactions in the mitochondria of the cell. The many reactions of the aerobic system include aerobic glycolysis, the Krebs cycle and the electron transport system. The initial stage is the same as with the previous system as glycogen is broken down to pyruvic acid but when oxygen is available lactic acid does not accumulate as the breakdown of pyruvic acid continues. It is chemically altered enabling it to enter the Krebs cycle and the electron transport system where the breakdown continues to yield carbon dioxide, water and energy (ATP).

This system provides far more energy than the other two systems as 1 molecule of glycogen will provide enough energy to resynthesise 38 moles of ATP. This system will therefore provide a continual supply of energy for prolonged endurance activities without producing fatiguing by-products. The activity can continue indefinitely providing the supply of oxygen and the fuel stores can be maintained. This system utilises both carbohydrate and fat as fuel but protein will only be used in extreme conditions of starvation or ultra marathon running.

Which system?

The systems used will depend on the intensity and duration of the activity. Most activities will utilise both anaerobic and aerobic systems depending on the availability of oxygen. However, as a general rule, short bursts of fast intense activity will utilise the anaerobic systems while prolonged low intensity activity will utilise the aerobic system.

Which fuel?

The fuel used to resynthesise ATP is provided by digested nutrients which include carbohydrates, fats and proteins.

Carbohydrates are starches and sugars which are converted to glucose or glycogen and stored in the blood, liver and muscle tissue. Carbohydrates provide primary fast energy during short bursts of intense anaerobic activity and moderate aerobic activity. However, glycogen stores are limited and become depleted during prolonged activities. Acute feelings of exhaustion are experienced as glycogen is depleted, as in 'hitting the wall' in marathon running.

Fats in the form of fatty acids and triglycerides are stored in the liver and adipose tissue. Fats are the body's most concentrated source of energy. The body is able to store far more fat than glycogen and twice as much energy is stored in one gram of fat, than in one gram of carbohydrate. Therefore fats provide a far greater source of potential energy for prolonged endurance activities.

However, fat requires a small amount of glycogen for its combustion and if glycogen stores are depleted, fat cannot be broken down. Fat cannot provide energy for fast activity, because it depends on the availability of oxygen, which depends on a person's aerobic capacity. Training improves aerobic capacity and a fit person with a high aerobic capacity will burn fat more easily. During endurance activities, the sooner fat can be utilised, the more glycogen will be spared which will prolong activity.

Proteins are broken down to amino acids and are used for growth, body building and tissue repair. Proteins are only used as an energy source if stores of carbohydrates and fats are very low or depleted as in conditions of starvation.

Table 4.1
The three metabolic systems

Anaerobic (alactic): ATP-PC system	Anaerobic: lactic acid system	Aerobic: oxygen system
Uses stored ATP and PC	Uses glycogen	Uses glycogen, fatty acids, triglycerol
Beginning of all activities and very fast short bursts up to 10–15 seconds	Fast activity up to 2–3 minutes	Slow steady moderate to low intensity, long duration activity
Example: quick dash, sprint	Example: 400 metre run	Example: jogging, marathon running
Contraction stops when ATP and PC are used up	Contraction stops due to lack of oxygen and lactic acid build-up.	Contraction maintained indefinitely until glycogen is depleted and exhaustion is reached

Aerobic and anaerobic exercises

These names are derived from the energy systems used. Most activities involve both aerobic and anaerobic metabolism.

Aerobic exercises

These are endurance activities that utilise oxygen for energy production. They are slow, steady-state exercises, which allow for the systems to supply sufficient oxygen for the complete breakdown of glycogen. Oxygen supply is maintained throughout and no oxygen debt is incurred. There is therefore no gasping or deep breathing at the end of these activities. Aerobic activities include jogging, walking, swimming, cycling, aerobic classes. (Remember that if the exercises become too fast and vigorous in aerobic classes, the exercise will be anaerobic. Clients should not be short of breath during aerobic activities and should be able to talk or sing whilst exercising.)

Anaerobic exercises

These are activities that do not use oxygen for energy production. All activities begin anaerobically and continue until all readily available energy within the muscles is used up; this will last for 10–15 seconds, until supplies of ATP and PC are exhausted and is known as the *alactic phase*, as lactic acid is not produced. Further vigorous, fast-moving activities – too fast for the systems to supply oxygen – will result in the incomplete breakdown of glycogen and the breakdown of pyruvic acid into lactic acid. This is known as the *lactic phase*. Lactic acid builds up within the muscle and will eventually inhibit its contraction. Anaerobic activities include squash, sprinting, hurdling and fast vigorous actions. There will be deep breathing or panting at the end of this activity as extra oxygen is required to re-establish homeostasis (body balance).

Most sports utilise both energy systems, where the fast vigorous phases are anaerobic and the slower steadier phases are aerobic.

Oxygen uptake

Oxygen uptake is the amount of oxygen consumed within a certain time: usually one minute. It is known as VO_2. Maximum oxygen uptake is the maximum amount of oxygen taken in, transported and utilised by the muscles per minute to produce energy. The amount of oxygen consumed at rest is around 0.2–0.3 litres per minute, but this increases considerably during exercise, to a point where the system is unable to meet further demand. This point is an individual's *aerobic capacity* or *VO_2 maximum*.

VO_2 maximum can be measured and is used to assess a person's aerobic power or fitness. With training, fitness develops, the heart pumps out more blood, the lungs improve and ventilation increases, with more oxygen taken in. This in turn is delivered to the muscles and used more efficiently. As fitness increases the amount of oxygen taken in increases. Trained athletes have far higher VO_2 maxima than untrained individuals.

Regular training increases the capacity for oxygen uptake and the ability to exercise aerobically for longer periods.

Oxygen debt

This is the excess amount of oxygen taken in during recovery, over and above that normally consumed. As previously explained, during vigorous muscular activity, oxygen cannot be supplied fast enough to the muscle fibres and oxygen supplies are depleted. Energy is therefore generated from the anaerobic breakdown of pyruvic acid, which produces lactic acid. A large percentage of the lactic acid is transported from the muscle to the liver, where it is converted back to glucose or glycogen, but some lactic acid remains in the muscle. After exercise has stopped, extra oxygen is required to metabolise the lactic acid, and to replenish ATP, phosphocreatine and glycogen, as well as increasing the supply of oxygen in the blood and lungs in order to restore the body systems to their normal state. The increase of lactic acid and carbon dioxide in the blood stimulates the respiratory system, so that breathing increases in depth and rate and oxygen debt is repaid.

Muscle fatigue

Muscle fatigue is the inability of a muscle to sustain a contraction. The contraction becomes progressively weaker and then fails completely as the muscle is unable to produce sufficient energy to meet its needs. During fast, vigorous exercise it is thought to be due to a build up of lactic acid in the muscle and blood. During low intensity exercise it is thought to be due to depletion of glycogen and dehydration.

Muscular soreness

Two types of muscular soreness have been identified:
Acute muscular soreness and *delayed muscular soreness*.

Acute muscular soreness is experienced during or immediately following activity. It is thought that this is due to an insufficient blood supply to the contracting muscles. This may be due to the tension which builds up in the contracting muscles pressing on the blood vessels, reducing or occluding blood flow. Metabolic waste products such as lactic acid are not removed and built up within the muscle to such an extent that they stimulate the pain receptors within the muscle. This acute soreness is quickly relieved when exercise stops and blood flows freely again flushing out the lactic acid.

Delayed muscle soreness or delayed onset muscle soreness (DOMS)
The onset of this soreness is delayed for 24–48 hours after the activity. The exact cause is not known but it is thought that it may be due to damage of the tissues. This damage may include minor tears of the muscle fibres; damage of the connective tissue components within the muscle; or damage to tendons and ligaments through over stretching.

Another theory suggests that muscle spasm occurs; this exerts pressure on the blood vessels reducing blood flow, resulting in pain.

Stretching warm muscles before activity helps prevent soreness and stretching after the activity helps alleviate it. The stretches must be smooth and slow as any jerking or bounding might increase the damage.

Delayed muscular soreness is greatest following eccentric contraction, less following concentric contraction and least following isokinetic contraction (Chapter 6).

SKELETAL MUSCLE RESPONSE TO EXERCISE

The adaptations of skeletal muscle will depend on the type of activity undertaken.

Endurance training

■ Muscle endurance improves when a muscle is made to contract repeatedly against low or moderate resistance. As a result of endurance training other changes occur:

■ Increase in the number and size of blood vessels supplying blood to muscle fibres;

■ an increase in myoglobin content;

■ an increase in the density of the capillary networks supplying blood to muscle fibres;

■ an increase in the blood flow aided by blood shunting thus improving the delivery of oxygen and the removal of waste;

■ an increase in the size and number of mitochondria in the muscle cells, and therefore greater efficiency in utilising oxygen and generating energy stores;

■ an increase in glygocen stores. The increased availability of oxygen and glycogen raises the anaerobic threshold, so that the muscles use aerobic energy for longer periods, thus reducing levels of lactic acid. The muscles can continue contracting for longer periods without fatigue.

■ An increase in glycolitic and oxidative enzymes.

Strength training

■ Muscle strength will increase, providing the muscle is made to work against sub-maximal or maximal loads. As the muscle strengthens the load must be progressively increased.

■ More motor units are recruited, which increases the strength of contraction.

■ Muscle size (bulk) increases. Research to date suggests that this is due to the following adaptations:

■ an increase in the size and number of myofibrils

■ an increase in the contractile proteins myosin and actin

■ an increase in stored energy supplies (ATP, PC) and enzymes, giving a greater source of quick energy

■ an increase in connective tissue components.

Flexibility training

■ An increase in elasticity and extensibility of the muscle.

■ Neurological adaptation delaying the stretch reflex.

■ Flexibility exercises gently stretch connective tissue in the muscle and at a joint. Flexibility exercises performed before but particularly after an activity session will reduce muscle soreness.

Summary and aid to learning

Skeletal muscle forms the body flesh. Its functions are: to produce movement; to maintain posture; to generate heat; to stabilise joints.

It has three properties:

■ Contractability: it is able to contract

■ Extensibility: it is able to lengthen

■ Elasticity: it is able to return to its original length after being stretched.

Skeletal muscle cells are elongated fibres with many nuclei along their length. These fibres are grouped together into bundles called fasciculi. Many bundles arranged together form the muscle. The fibres, bundles and muscles are surrounded by 'sleeves' of connective tissue. This connective tissue blends together at the ends of the muscle to form the tendons.

Give the function of tendons.

When viewed under a powerful microscope light and dark bands can be seen along the length of the fibres. These are thick and thin filaments of the proteins, actin and myosin. It is the sliding of the thin actin filaments towards the thick myosin filaments that shortens the muscle, producing muscle contraction. This is known as the sliding filament theory.

There are two main types of muscle fibres within a muscle:
- Type I   Slow twitch, red fibres
- Type II   Fast twitch, white fibres

Study the text and write down six differences between these fibres.

Muscles are under the control of the nervous system, they contract in response to stimuli initiated in the brain.

The all or none law states that, *stimulated muscle fibres will contract with maximum force or not at all.*

Muscle tone – this is the state of partial contraction found in a muscle even at rest.

Sensory receptors within the muscles, known as *muscle spindles*, register the degree of stretch within a muscle.

The energy for muscle contraction is obtained from the breakdown of a chemical compound called adenosine triphosphate (ATP). All cells require ATP to carry out their functions but muscle cells require large amounts to maintain muscle contraction during exercise.

Only a small amount of ATP is stored in muscle cells, therefore when this is used up it must be continually remade (resynthesised). It is resynthesised from another chemical called phospho-creatine (PC) and from the food we eat, mainly carbohydrates and fats in the form of glycogen and triglycerides.

Therefore the energy for muscle contraction comes from stored ATP and from the other chemical reactions or systems which resynthesise it from foods. Some of the systems utilise oxygen and are known as aerobic systems while others do not need oxygen and are called anaerobic systems.

Remember: **aerobic means with oxygen**
             anaerobic means without oxygen

There are three systems which provide the energy for muscle contraction:

■ ATP – PC system uses stored ATP, PC, *anaerobic*.

■ Lactic acid system involves the incomplete breakdown of glycogen, *anaerobic*, and as its name suggests, lactic acid is produced which builds up in the muscle.

■ Aerobic system involves the complete breakdown of glycogen and triglycerides in the presence of oxygen, *aerobic*, carbon dioxide and water are produced.

The system used will depend on the intensity and duration of the activity.

Study the text and answer the following:

■ Which system would be used during marathon running and why?

■ Explain the main factor which limits contraction when very fast activity is performed.

Aerobic power (VO$_2$ maximum) is the maximal rate that an individual can take in and utilise oxygen during maximal performance. It is an indicator of cardiorespiratory fitness.

Oxygen debt or **recovery oxygen** is the amount of oxygen consumed after exercise, over and above that normally consumed. It is the amount of oxygen required to resynthesise ATP and PC stores in the muscle and to restore homeostasis.

Muscle fatigue is the inability of a muscle to sustain a contraction. The contraction becomes weaker and weaker and then fails completely. During fast, high intensity exercise, it is thought to be due to the build up of lactic acid in the muscles and the blood. During low intensity exercises it is thought to be caused mainly by depletion of glycogen, and dehydration.

Muscle soreness there are two types:

■ *acute muscular soreness* – this occurs immediately after performance;

■ *delayed muscular soreness or delayed onset muscular soreness DOMS*. This occurs 24–48 hours after performance.

Read the text and discuss the different causes of the two types of muscular soreness.

QUESTIONS

1. Give three functions of muscle tissue.
2. Name the connective tissue sheath which surrounds a muscle.
3. Name two contractile proteins found in muscle fibres.
4. Complete the following sentence: Muscle contraction occurs as a result of a stimulus from the … .
5. Explain what happens to a muscle fibre if no cross-bridges remain intact.
6. Name two types of muscle fibre.
7. State which type of muscle fibre depends on aerobic metabolism and which type depends on anaerobic metabolism.
8. Explain what is meant by the term *threshold stimulus*.
9. List any three factors which affect the strength of muscle contraction.
10. Define the following:
    a tendon
    b aponeurosis
    c origin
    d insertion.
11. Define the term *muscle tone*.
12. Name the structures which transmit information on the degree of tension found in a muscle.
13. Name the chemical which supplies energy for muscle contraction.
14. Briefly explain why energy is supplied by anaerobic metabolism for the first fifteen to twenty seconds of muscular activity.
15. Explain why lactic acid is produced during short, vigorous bursts of activity.
16. Explain the term *oxygen debt*.
17. State what types of exercise and activities utilise aerobic metabolism.
18. Differentiate between aerobic and anaerobic exercises.
19. Explain what is meant by the term VO_2 *maximum*.
20. Define the term *muscle fatigue* and explain how it occurs.

Chapter 5
The Support Systems: Nervous, Cardio-vascular and Respiratory

THE NERVOUS SYSTEM

The nervous system is the communication and control system of the body. It works with the endocrine system to maintain homeostasis (body balance). The nervous system will sense changes, interpret them and initiate appropriate action.

The nervous system is made up of:
1 *The central nervous system* comprising the brain and spinal cord which controls both reflex and voluntary movements. Here, incoming stimuli are processed, information is stored, thoughts are initiated and motor skills (movements) are controlled.
2 *The peripheral nervous system* comprising 12 pairs of cranial nerves arising from the brain and 31 pairs of spinal nerves arising from the spinal cord. These nerves conduct impulses from sensory organs to the spinal cord and brain and conduct impulses from the brain and spinal cord to muscles and glands.
3 *The autonomic system* comprising both sympathetic and parasympathetic parts which exercise involuntary control of body functions.

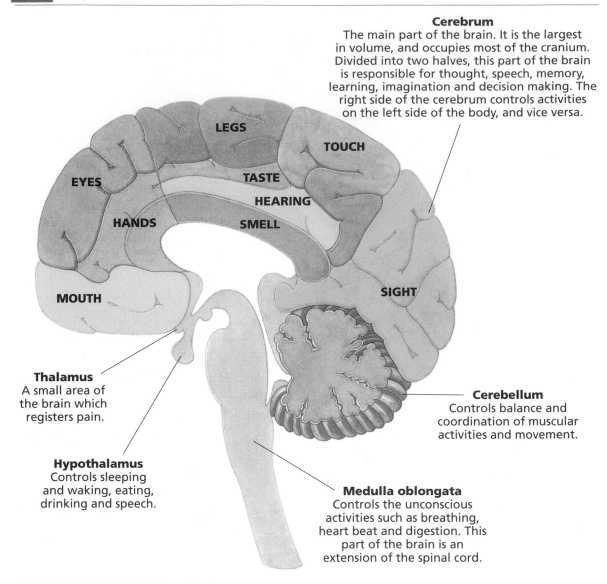

Cerebrum
The main part of the brain. It is the largest in volume, and occupies most of the cranium. Divided into two halves, this part of the brain is responsible for thought, speech, memory, learning, imagination and decision making. The right side of the cerebrum controls activities on the left side of the body, and vice versa.

LEGS

TOUCH

EYES

TASTE

HEARING

HANDS

SMELL

MOUTH

SIGHT

Thalamus
A small area of the brain which registers pain.

Cerebellum
Controls balance and coordination of muscular activities and movement.

Hypothalamus
Controls sleeping and waking, eating, drinking and speech.

Medulla oblongata
Controls the unconscious activities such as breathing, heart beat and digestion. This part of the brain is an extension of the spinal cord.

FIGURE NUMBER: 5.1 – The brain.

The autonomic system conducts information from the viscera to the central nervous system and information from the brain to smooth muscle, cardiac muscle and glands. This part is involuntary as it is not under conscious control.

Structure of the neurone

Nervous tissue is composed of the functional units which conduct impulses called *neurones* and the supporting tissue called *neuroglia*. There are three types of neurones:

■ Sensory neurones which transmit stimuli from sensory organs to the spinal cord and brain.

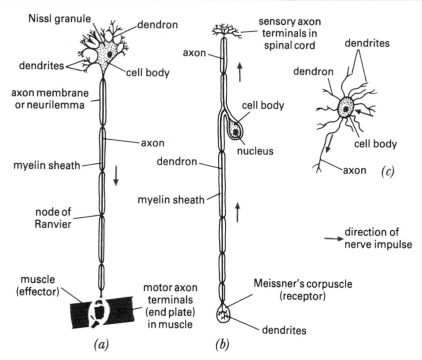

FIGURE NUMBER: 5.2 – Types of neurone. (a) Motorneurone. (b) Sensoryneurone.
(c) Interneurone.

■ Motor neurones which transmit stimuli from the brain and spinal cord to muscles and glands.
■ Inter-neurones which form a connection between neurones.

All neurones have a similar structure: they have a **cell body**, one long nerve fibre called an **axon** and several short nerve fibres called dendrons ending in dendrites.
■ Axons carry impulses *away* from the cell body.
■ Dendrons and dendrites carry impulses *towards* the cell body.

The axons of some nerves are protected by a fatty myeline sheath; this sheath is interrupted at intervals by small spaces called nodes of Ranvier. These determine the speed at which the nerve impulse is transmitted.

The nerve impulse

A nerve impulse is electrical in nature. It is generated in response to a stimulus and is transmitted along a nerve fibre due to changes in its electrically charged state. Impulses are transmitted in axons and dendrons in one direction only. The fatty myeline sheath insulates parts of the nerve and the impulse must jump from one node of Ranvier to another. This jumping from node to node serves to increase the speed of transmission.

Synapses

The point of connection between the axon of one nerve cell and the dendrites or body of another is known as a **synapse**. This is a gap across which the impulse must be relayed. When an impulse reaches a synapse, a chemical transmitter is released which facilitates or inhibits the passage of the impulse across the gap. The chemical transmitters at a synapse may be excitatory transmitters such as acetylcholine (ACh) which facilitates the passage of the impulse across the gap or it may be an inhibitory transmitter such as gamma-aminobutyric acid (GABA) which will inhibit its passage.

The point at which a nerve connects with its muscle fibre is known as the neuromuscular junction. It is similar in structure to a synapse. However, all stimuli are transmitted across this junction by the transmitter acetylcholine (ACh) as there is no inhibitory chemical transmitter here. The acetylcholine initiates an action potential in the muscle and the muscle contracts.

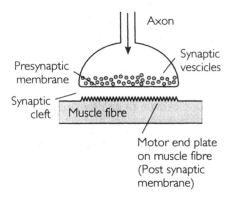

FIGURE NUMBER: 5.3 – Synapse between nerve terminal and muscle fibre.

Muscle sense organs

There are several types of sense organs in muscles. These include **pain receptors** which are found in muscle fibres, in the connective tissue components of muscles and in the walls of the arteries which supply the muscles. These register pain or soreness when a muscle is worked too vigorously or sustains injury.

Other kinds of sense organs are called **proprioceptors** which conduct sensory reports from muscle, tendons, ligaments and joints. These enable us to execute smooth co-ordinated movement. Three important muscle sense organs are: muscle spindles, Golgi tendon organs and joint receptors.

Muscle spindles, also known as stretch receptors, are found within special muscle fibres. They provide the CNS with information regarding the degree of stretch within the muscle. If there is too much stretch, which may result in damage to the muscle, more motor units are recruited to strengthen the contraction and shorten the muscle.

Golgi tendon organs are located in tendon fibres near the junction between the tendon and the muscle. They are also sensitive to stretch and are stretched when the muscle in whose tendon they lie contracts. When the contraction is too strong the stretch in the GTO is relayed to the CNS causing the contracted muscle to relax. This protects the muscle from injury.

Joint receptors are found in tendons, ligaments, joint capsules and in the periostium covering bones. They provide information concerning joint position and angle and together with other reflexes are concerned with the maintenance of posture.

Neuromuscular control

The selection and performance of motor movement is initiated in the motor cortex of the brain. The primary motor area is subdivided according to body areas and is responsible for specific patterns of movement, while the pre-motor area is responsible for more complex patterns; this is also called the sports skill area. The three areas of the brain most involved in the execution of movement are the cerebral cortex, basal ganglia, and cerebellum. Impulses are transmitted from the brain via the upper motor neurone to the anterior horn of the spinal cord. Here the impulse will cross a synapse to stimulate the lower motor neurone and will be transmitted via its axon to the muscle fibres, resulting in contraction of the muscle. Information from the sense organs will be transmitted back to the brain regarding the spatial location of body parts. etc., and the degree of stretch in muscles and tendons. The other areas of the brain such as the cerebellum and basal ganglia are responsible for synchronising actions and with the execution of smooth, co-ordinated movement. Training and practice reinforces patterns of movement in the brain and has a positive effect on reflex action and on the transmission of impulses. As a result, skill, co-ordination, balance, rhythm, timing and reaction will improve.

Summary and aid to learning

The nervous system is a communication and control system.

The nervous system is made up of:
- *central nervous system* composed of the brain and spinal cord.
- *peripheral nervous system* comprising 12 pairs of cranial nerves and 31 pairs of spinal nerves.
- *autonomic nervous system* comprising the sympathetic and parasympathetic parts.

Nerve cells are called neurones; there are three types:
- *Sensory neurones*
- *Motor neurones*
- *Inter neurones*

Explain the function of each type.

A *synapse* is the point of connection between two neurones – it is a gap across which the impulses must be transmitted.

The chemical acetylcholine facilitates the passage of the impulse across the gap. The chemical gamma-aminobutyric acid will inhibit its passage.

The point of connection between a nerve fibre and a muscle fibre is known as the *neuro-muscular junction*. It is similar in structure to a synapse but only acetylcholine is released here.

The point where the nerve enters the muscle is known as the *motor point*. The point on the muscle fibre where the nerve connects is known as the *motor end plate*.

There are sense organs within a muscle which register pain or soreness. There are also stretch receptors which register the degree of stretch within the muscle; these are the *muscle spindles*.

Name the sensory receptors found in tendons and explain their function.

The nervous system initiates and coordinates movement during exercise.

THE CARDIO-VASCULAR SYSTEM (BLOOD CIRCULATORY SYSTEM)

The cardio-vascular system is a closed circuit. It is composed of a pump, called the heart, a network of inter-connecting tubes, called blood vessels, and the fluid which flows through them, called blood.

The system is designed to carry oxygenated blood to the cells and to take away deoxygenated blood from the cells. (Oxygenated blood contains oxygen, nutrients, hormones, enzymes, etc., while deoxygenated blood contains carbon dioxide and the waste products of metabolism.)

Parts of the cardio-vascular system
- The heart
- Arteries and arterioles
- Capillaries
- Veins and venules
- Blood

All the body cells are bathed in interstitial fluid (tissue fluid). This fluid provides the medium for substances to move in and out of the cells and capillaries. Oxygenated blood flows from the heart, through the arteries and arterioles to the capillaries. The walls of the capillaries are very thin, consequently the oxygen and nutrients easily pass out through the walls into the interstitial fluid and then into the cells.

The waste products of metabolism (metabolites) pass out through the cell walls into the tissue fluid and then into the capillaries in the same way. They are then transported in the deoxygenated blood via the venules and veins back to the heart. The heart then pumps this

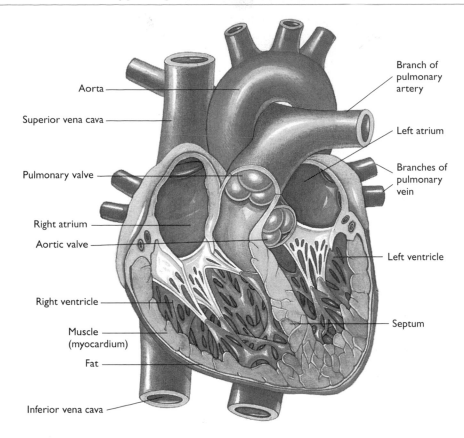

Aorta

Superior vena cava

Pulmonary valve

Right atrium

Aortic valve

Right ventricle

Muscle
(myocardium)

Fat

Inferior vena cava

Branch of
pulmonary
artery

Left atrium

Branches of
pulmonary
vein

Left ventricle

Septum

FIGURE NUMBER: 5.4 – The heart.

deoxygenated blood to the lungs to be reoxygenated. The passage of substances across the cell membranes and blood vessel walls is controlled by differences in pressure on each side of the wall or membrane.

The structure of the heart

The heart is a muscular organ and contains four chambers. The heart lies in the thoracic cavity between the lungs. It is about 12cm in length, and weighs 250–350 grams. It is somewhat cone shaped, having a base above and an apex below. It lies to the left of mid-line, approximately two-thirds to the left and one-third to the right. It is protected on each side by the lungs; in front by the sternum; below by the diaphragm. It also further protected by the rib cage and chest muscles.

The wall of the heart

This is composed of three layers of tissue: the pericardium, the myocardium and the endocardium.

- The *pericardium* is the tough outer coat, which is composed of an outer sac of tough fibrous tissue lined with a double layer of serous membrane. This serous membrane secretes serous fluid which lubricates, reduces friction and allows smooth movement as the heart beats.

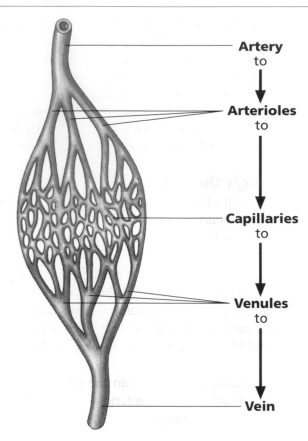

Artery
to
↓
Arterioles
to
↓
Capillaries
to
↓
Venules
to
↓
Vein

FIGURE NUMBER: 5.5 – Blood flow from artery to vein.

- The *myocardium* is the middle muscular coat, composed of specialised muscle tissue found only in the heart called *cardiac muscle*. It is thinnest around the base and atria and thickest around the apex and ventricles.
- The *endocardium* is the inner lining. This is a smooth membrane of simple squamous epithelial cells. It is continuous with the lining of the blood vessels.

The interior of the heart

The heart is divided into right and left sides by a muscular septum. The left side of the heart deals with oxygenated blood while the right side deals with deoxygenated blood. Each side of the heart is further divided into two chambers separated by valves.

The upper chambers are called the **atria** (singular atrium). The lower chambers are called the **ventricles**. One-way valves divide the atria and ventricles. The valve dividing the right atrium and right ventricle is called the *tricuspid* valve and is made up of three flaps or cusps. The valve dividing the left atrium and left ventricle is called the *bicuspid* valve (or *mitral* valve) and is made up of two flaps or cusps. These valves allow the blood to flow in one direction only – from the atria into the ventricles. They open and close as a result of changes in pressure within the chambers.

When the atria become full of blood and contract, the pressure increases and the valves open, and blood flows into the ventricles. When the ventricles contract, the pressure increases and blood is pumped into the arteries. Backward flow into the atria is prevented because the tricuspid and bicuspid valves close. The valves are held in place by cords attached to the under surface of the cusps and the walls of the ventricles. These cords are called the *chordae tendineae*. They are attached to the ventricle walls by small muscles – the *papillary muscles*. Both the arteries that leave the heart, i.e. the *pulmonary artery* from the right ventricle and the *aorta* from the left ventricle, also have one-way valves to prevent backward flow. These are known as *semi-lunar* valves.

The flow of blood through the heart

- Deoxygenated blood from all the body tissues flows via the *inferior vena cava, the superior vena cava* and *coronary sinus* into the right atrium. At the same time oxygenated blood from the lungs flows via the pulmonary vein into the left atrium. The atria then contract.

- Blood from the right atrium then passes through the *tricuspid valve* into the right ventricle and from the left atrium through the *bicuspid valve* into the left ventricle. Then the ventricles contract pushing the semi-lunar valves open.

- Blood from the right ventricle is pumped into the *pulmonary artery* (the only artery carrying deoxygenated blood) and taken to the lungs where the interchange of gases occurs.

- Blood from the left ventricle is pumped into the *aorta* – this artery divides and sub-divides into numerous smaller arteries, arterioles and capillaries which carry oxygenated blood to all the cells in the body.

Cardiac blood supply

The heart is mainly muscle tissue and requires its own blood supply to provide it with oxygen and to remove waste products. The blood supply to the heart is known as the **coronary circulation**.

The right and left coronary arteries branch off the aorta and carry oxygenated blood and nutrients to cardiac muscle cells.

The deoxygenated blood is collected in the coronary vein then drains into the *coronary sinus*, which empties directly into the right atrium. Any problems or blockages developing in the coronary circulation will reduce the oxygen supply to the cells. The cells may be weakened and fail to function efficiently resulting in a condition called *ischemia*, and giving rise to chest pains known as *angina pectoris*. If the blood supply is completely cut off to an area of heart muscle due to a thrombus or embolus, the tissue dies and the heart muscle loses some of its strength; this is known as a *heart attack*. This will cause distress and if the damage is extensive, may result in death.

Summary
Right side
Inferior and superior venae cavae and coronary sinus (deoxygenated)
   into

right atrium then through tricuspid valve
  into
Right ventricle
  into
Pulmonary artery – to lungs

Left side
Pulmonary vein from lungs (oxygenated)
  into
Left atrium then through bicuspid valve
  into
Left ventricle
  into
the aorta and via branching arteries on to tissue cells.

Blood vessels

These are tubes through which blood flows. There are three types of blood vessels, namely arteries, veins and capillaries.

Arteries

Transport blood away from the heart. Arteries carry oxygenated blood, nutrients, etc., to the cells, with the exception of the pulmonary artery, which carries deoxygenated blood from the heart to the lungs. Artery walls are composed of three layers of tissue. These layers surround a hollow core called a *lumen*.

The outer layer is fibrous tissue with elastin and collagen.

The middle layer is *smooth* muscular tissue.

The inner layer is simple squamous epithelium called *endothelium*.

As the heart pumps blood into the arteries, they expand to accommodate the blood, then, as the heart relaxes, the artery walls recoil propelling the blood forwards.

Arteries leaving and near the heart are large, but these branch and become smaller until they become small arterioles with thinner walls.

Veins

Veins transport blood back to the heart. The walls of the veins are similar in structure to those of the arteries, except that the outer layer is thicker and the middle muscular layer is thinner. The inner layer endothelium folds to form valves. These valves prevent the backward flow of blood. The lumen of the veins is larger. Veins carry deoxygenated blood and waste products from cells back to the heart, except for the pulmonary vein, which carries oxygenated blood from the lungs to the heart. Blood flows back from the cells to the right side of the heart and is known as *venous return*. Venous return is helped along the veins by the contraction and relaxation of muscles and by the expansion and contraction of the thorax and diaphragm during breathing; these actions are known as 'the muscle pump' and 'the respiratory pump'. If the muscles are not contracting, e.g. during long periods of standing or inactivity, gravity exerts a downward force on the blood. If the valves are weak this pressure overloads the vein and the wall bulges outwards causing the condition known as 'varicose veins'. If exercise stops suddenly blood pools in the legs depleting the supply to the brain which can result in dizziness and fainting. The very small veins at the capillary end are known as venules.

Capillaries

These are tiny vessels connecting arterioles and venules. The walls of the capillaries are very thin, composed of a single layer of squamous epithelium (endothelium). Capillaries form networks among tissue cells with arterioles leading into them and venules leading away. The primary function of capillaries is to allow exchange of gases, nutrients and waste products between the cells and the blood. When metabolic needs are low, part of the network can shut off and blood flows through a small portion only of the capillary network. When metabolic needs are high, the networks dilate increasing blood flow. As activity increases, there will be an increase in demand for nutrients and oxygen by the contracting muscles, hence the blood vessels and capillaries in the muscles dilate but at the same time the vessels and capillaries in other organs such as the stomach, kidneys and liver constrict, so that extra blood is delivered to the muscles. This is known as ***blood shunting***.

Blood

Blood is a liquid connective tissue which performs many functions. It is a viscous (slightly sticky) fluid which flows through the heart and blood vessels. Its temperature is around 38°C and its pH is around 7.4 (slightly alkaline). The total volume of blood in the human body is around 5½ litres (5–6 litres in men and 4–5 litres in women).

It is composed of a faintly yellow transparent fluid known as *plasma* which contains dissolved substances and different types of cells.
- 55 percent of the total volume is plasma.
- 45 percent of the total volume is cells.

Plasma

A straw-coloured transparent fluid composed of approximately 91 percent water, 7 percent proteins and 2 percent other solutes.

Substances found in plasma:
1 Plasma proteins: albumin, globulin, fibrinogen and prothrombin (important for blood clotting).
2 Mineral salts (electrolytes): sodium, potassium, magnesium, phosphorus, calcium, etc.
3 Dissolved foods (nutrients): amino acids, fatty acids, glycerol glucose and vitamins.

4   Hormones produced by endocrine glands.
5   Enzymes secreted by specialised cells.
6   Gases: oxygen, carbon dioxide, etc.
7   Antibodies and antitoxins.
8   Waste products of metabolism: urea, uric acid, etc.

Blood cells

There are 3 main types of cells in blood:

1   Erythrocytes – red blood cells; these contain haemoglobin, whose function is the transportation of oxygen from the lungs to body cells and carbon dioxide from cells to the lungs.
2   Leucocytes – white blood cells; there are many types. They are phagocytic cells i.e. they destroy and ingest micro-organisms thus protecting the body against infection and disease.
3   Platelets or throbocytes – these play an important role in preventing blood loss. They initiate a chain of reactions resulting in blood clotting.

Functions of blood

1   It *transports* substances around the body.
   i   Oxygen from the lungs to body cells, mainly by combining with haemoglobin in the blood, to form oxyhaemoglobin. The concentration of haemoglobin in the blood increases through endurance training.
   ii   Carbon dioxide from cells to the lungs: some is transported by combining with haemoglobin but most is transported in the form of bicarbonate ions.
   iii Nutrients from digestive tract to body cells.
   iv   Metabolic waste products from cells to excretory organs.
   v   Hormones from endocrine glands to the cells.
   vi   Any drugs taken for medicinal purposes.
2   It *regulates:*
   i   The water content of cells.
   ii   Body heat, maintaining normal body temperature.
   iii pH by means of buffers.
3   It protects
   i   Against disease and infection through lencocytes, destroying micro-organisms, phagocytic action and production of antibodies.
   ii   Against blood loss by the process of blood clotting.

Conduction system of the heart

The beating of the heart is under the influence of the autonomic nervous system which controls the strength and rate of contraction. The sympathetic nervous system increases heart rate and the parasympathetic slows it down. These are regulated by the cardio-acceleratory centre and the cardio-inhibitory centres of the medulla which respond to variations in blood pressure, to the concentration of chemicals in the blood and to temperature variations.

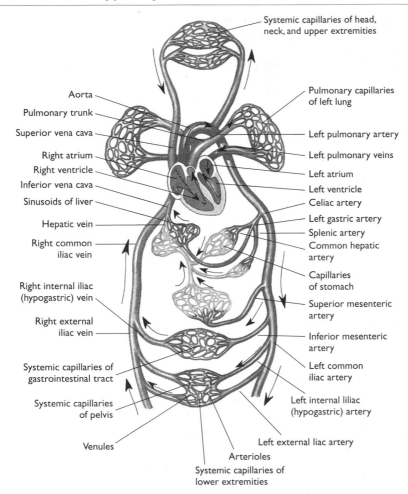

Systemic capillaries of head, neck, and upper extremities

Aorta

Pulmonary trunk

Superior vena cava

Right atrium

Right ventricle

Inferior vena cava

Sinusoids of liver

Hepatic vein

Right common iliac vein

Right internal iliac (hypogastric) vein

Right external iliac vein

Systemic capillaries of gastrointestinal tract

Systemic capillaries of pelvis

Venules

Arterioles

Systemic capillaries of lower extremities

Pulmonary capillaries of left lung

Left pulmonary artery

Left pulmonary veins

Left atrium

Left ventricle

Celiac artery

Left gastric artery

Splenic artery

Common hepatic artery

Capillaries of stomach

Superior mesenteric artery

Inferior mesenteric artery

Left common iliac artery

Left internal liliac (hypogastric) artery

Left external liliac artery

FIGURE NUMBER: 5.6 – The circulatory system.

However, the heart will contract and relax without a direct stimulus from the nervous system as the heart muscle has its own built in conduction system. Contraction is initiated in specialised tissue called the sino-atrial (SA) node (known as the pacemaker) found in the wall of the right atrium. From here, impulses spread throughout the atria resulting in their contraction. They then pass to the atrio-ventricular (AV) node found in the right atrium (at the atrio-ventricule junction) and then on to the Purkinge fibres. These are specialised fibres which spread the impulse throughout the ventricles resulting in their contraction. The movement of blood through the heart occurs as a result of changes in pressure between the atria and ventricles.

The cardiac cycle

The cardiac cycle refers to the electrical and mechanical changes that occur in the heart during and following a single heart beat. When the heart is beating normally the cardiac cycle occurs about 74 times every minute. Thus each cycle lasts for 0.8 of a second.

- The term *systole* is used for the contraction time.
- The term *diastole* is used for the relaxation time.
1 Atrial systole – contraction of the atria for 0.1 of a second.
2 Atrial diastole – relaxation of the atria for 0.7 of a second.
3 Ventricular systole – contraction of the ventricles for 0.3 of a second.
4 Ventricular diastole – relaxation of the ventricles of 0.5 of a second.
   (The sum of atrial and ventricular systole is 0.4 of a second therefore the heart is totally relaxed for 0.4 of a second.)

The superior and inferior vena cavae pour blood into the right atrium; at the same time the pulmonary veins pour blood into the left atrium. The SA node sends an impulse to contract and the atria contract for 0.1 of a second and blood is pushed through the valves into the ventricles. The AV node sends an impulse to contract and the ventricles contract for 0.3 of a second. Blood is pushed by the right ventricle into the pulmonary artery and by the left ventricle into the aorta. After contraction of the ventricles the heart rests for 0.4 of a second then the cycle begins again.

Cardiac output

Cardiac output is the amount of blood ejected per minute from the left ventricle of the heart. It is a product of stroke volume and heart rate.

Stroke volume is the amount of blood ejected by the left ventricle during one contraction or systole (average stroke volume in the adult is around 70 ml).

Heart rate is the number of beats/minute (average is around 74 beats/min).

Cardiac output is calculated as follows:
cardiac output = stroke volume × heart rate (number of beats/min)

Therefore using average values
cardiac output = 70 ml × 74/min
                = 5180 ml/min or 5.2 litres/min.

Blood pressure

This is the force or pressure which the blood exerts on the walls of the blood vessels in which it is contained. The blood pressure in the arteries is higher than that in the veins. The arterial blood pressure is the result of the left ventricle pushing blood into the aorta. This pressure is known as systolic blood pressure and is found to be around 120 mmHg (millimetres of mercury). During complete cardiac diastole, i.e. the heart resting, the blood pressure falls to around 80 mmHg. These figures vary depending on the individual, the degree of activity and the time of day – it tends to be lower at rest.

It is measured using a SPHYGMOMANOMETER and expressed BP $= \dfrac{120}{80}$ mmHg.

Factors affecting normal blood pressure (BP)

1 Cardiac output: the amount of blood ejected by the left ventricle into the aorta affects blood pressure. An increase in cardiac output raises blood pressure while a decrease in cardiac output lowers blood pressure.

2 Volume of blood: enough blood must be circulating through the system (normally around $5\frac{1}{2}$ litres) to maintain normal BP. Blood loss during haemorrhage reduces quantity of blood flowing in the system and blood pressure drops. If the blood volume increases the blood pressure increases.

3 Peripheral resistance: BP varies with constriction and dilation of the arterioles known as vaso-dilation and vasoconstriction. Constriction of arterioles raises BP, dilation of arterioles lowers BP (remember this happens when the body is heated).

4 Elasticity of the arterial walls – the amount of stretch and recoil of the arterial walls affects BP.

The pulse rate

The pulse rate is the same as the heart rate, being around 74 beats/min. The pulse can be felt because of the expansion and elastic recoil of the arteries during each ventricular systole (contraction). The pulse is strongest in the arteries closest to the heart. The pulse is usually taken at the radial artery at the wrist but can be taken at the carotid artery in the neck or the brachial artery, medial to the biceps muscle.

The clotting or coagulation of blood

When a blood vessel is damaged blood will escape. To prevent blood loss the body reacts by a mechanism called clotting or coagulation of blood. It is a very complex process. Certain substances must be present for clotting to occur. They are:

> Prothrombin ⎫ These three substances
> Calcium ⎬ are always present
> Fibrinogen ⎭ in the blood.
> and
> Thromboplastin which is only released from damaged thrombocytes when injury occurs.

Stages of blood clotting

When bleeding starts the release of *Thromboplastin* triggers a series of reactions which end with the formation of a blood clot. In a simplified form the stages are as follows:

Prothrombin acted on by Thromboplastin in the presence of calcium will be converted into Thrombin. Thrombin then acts upon Fibrinogen which is converted into threads of fibrin. These fibrin threads form a mesh which together with trapped blood cells result in a blockage or clot which stops further bleeding. After a time the clot shrinks and dries as serum is released and healing takes place. (The drug Heparin is an anti-coagulant which prevents prothrombin being converted to thrombin.)

Cardio-vascular response to exercise

As previously discussed in chapter 4, muscle contraction is dependent on ATP, which is the energy source for all cellular activity. Once exercise begins, the small quantity of ATP stored in muscle cells is quickly used up. If contraction continues, ATP must be resynthesised using glycogen from liver stores and oxygen from the lungs. These are transported to the muscles via the blood. Hence the cardio-vascular system must quickly respond to this increased demand for oxygen and glycogen by the contracting muscles and the following changes occur.

- The heart rate increases dramatically, from around 80 beats/min to 180 beats/min.
- The heart pumps out a larger volume of blood per beat (stroke volume).
- The cardiac output therefore increases greatly, from around 5–6 L/min at rest to around 30 L/min during maximal activity.
- Changes in blood pressure depend on the type of exercises. During aerobic exercises, systolic pressure increases as a result of cardiac output, but diastolic pressure remains constant. During anaerobic and isometric exercises, both systolic and diastolic pressure rises, due to pressure on, and resistance of, the blood vessels.
- Blood flow to the muscles and other organs changes once exercise commences. At rest, only 15–20 percent of cardiac output is transported to skeletal muscle. However, during intense exercise this may go up to around 80 percent of cardiac output as blood is redirected from the other organs such as the stomach, liver and kidneys to the exercising muscles. This is controlled by vasoconstriction and vasodilation of the arterioles and is known as *blood shunting*.

After a period of training there will be further adaptations:
- The heart increases in size and volume.
- The muscular wall of the heart becomes thicker.
- More blood flows into the left ventricle; this contracts more forcefully pumping a larger volume of blood around the body.
- The resting heart rate decreases: because the heart pumps out more blood with each beat, fewer beats per minute are necessary. Endurance athletes may have heart rates as low as 40 beats per minute.
- There is an increase in the size and number of blood vessels and in the density of capillary networks in the heart and in the muscles. This improves the delivery of oxygen and nutrients and speeds up the removal of waste.
- There is an increase in the haemoglobin content of the blood which increases its oxygen carrying capacity.

The functions of the blood during exercise are:
- To transport oxygen from the lungs to the contracting muscles
- To transport carbon dioxide from the muscles to the lungs
- To transport lactic acid from the muscles to the liver
- To transport glucose from the liver stores to the muscles
- To regulate body temperature by transporting heat to the surface
- To maintain body homeostasis, i.e. body equilibrium.

Summary and aid to learning

The function of the cardio-vascular system is the transportation of substances around the body.

The cardio-vascular system is composed of the heart, arteries, arterioles, capillaries, veins, venules and blood.

The heart has four chambers: right and left atrium, right and left ventricles.

The right side of the heart deals with deoxygenated blood.

The left side deals with oxygenated blood.

Structure

The wall of the heart is made up of three coats or layers.
1 Pericardium – tough outer coat of fibrous tissue lined with serous membrane, lubricated for smooth movement.
2 Myocardium – middle muscular coat, special muscle tissue called cardiac muscle.
3 Endocardium – inner smooth coat of squamous epithelium.

The heart tissue is supplied with blood via the coronary circulation.

Valves of the heart
1 Tricuspid valve has three flaps and divides the right atrium and right ventricle.
2 Bicuspid (Mital) valve has two flaps and divides the left atrium and left ventricle.
3 Semi-lunar valves are found at the openings of the arteries, the aorta on the left and the pulmonary artery on the right.

Blood Vessels of the Heart

Inferior and superior venae cavae and coronary sinus enter the right atrium (deoxygenated).

Pulmonary vein enters the left atrium (oxygenated).

Pulmonary artery leaves the right ventricle (deoxygenated).

Aorta leaves the left ventricle (oxygenated).

Venous return

This is the deoxygenated blood carried from the tissues back to the heart. It is aided by the muscle pump – contraction of muscles, and the respiratory pump – movement of thorax and contraction of diaphragm.

Blood Vessels

There are three types: arteries, veins, capillaries.

1 Arteries carry oxygenated blood away from the heart (except the pulmonary artery).
2 Veins carry deoxygenated blood to the heart (except the pulmonary vein).
3 Capillaries – thin walled vessels which form networks throughout tissue spaces and allow interchange of gases, nutrients and waste products. Arteries branch and become smaller arterioles; these enter into the capillaries, venules leave capillaries and join to form veins.

Blood

A viscous fluid; temperature 38°C; pH 7.4; volume 5–6 litres in males, 4–5 litres in females. Blood is composed of 55 percent plasma and 45 percent cells.

Plasma is straw coloured, composed of 91 percent water, 7 percent proteins, 2 percent other solutes.

The blood transports substances around the body; regulates water content, body heat and pH; it protects against disease and blood loss.

List the substances transported by the blood.
Blood cells: three main types

1 Erythrocytes – red blood cells contain haemoglobin which transports oxygen and carbon dioxide.
2 Leucocycytes – white blood cells, many types protect the body against micro-organisms.
3 Thrombocytes or platelets play an important role in blood clotting.

Cardiac cycle: systole is the contraction phase, diastole the relaxation phase.

The cardiac cycle occurs about 74 times per minute, each cycle taking 0.8 of a second.

Cardiac output is the amount of blood ejected into the aorta every minute; it is the product of stroke volume x beats per minute.

Pulse rate – this is the same as heart rate, the average being 74/min.

Blood pressure is the force exerted on the walls of arteries.

> systolic pressure 120 mmHg
> diastolic pressure 80 mmHg.

Blood clotting

Thromboplastin released from damaged throbocytes acts on Prothrombin in the presence of calcium, converting it to Thrombin; this acts on fibrinogen converting it into threads of fibrin. These threads form a mesh with released blood cells forming a scab/clot which covers and seals the wound, preventing further blood loss.

Main circulatory routes are:

1 The Systemic or General circulation to the body, heart and brain.
2 The Pulmonary circulation to the lungs.
3 The Portal circulation to the liver.

The heart plays a major role during exercise because the cardio-vascular system must increase the delivery of oxygen to the contracting muscles and increase the speed of removal of waste products. In response to regular exercise the heart will improve in strength and function.

Study the text and write a list of the changes and improvements found in the cardio-vascular system following regular training.

THE RESPIRATORY SYSTEM

This system is responsible for the exchange of oxygen and carbon dioxide between the external environment and the internal environment of the body. It is closely linked with the cardio-vascular system as the exchange of gases takes place between the alveoli of the lungs and the blood in the pulmonary capillaries.

The system is composed of:
- The nose and nasal passages
- The pharynx
- The larynx
- The trachea
- The bronchi and bronchioles
- The lungs which are composed of alveoli.

The nose

The nose serves as the first section of the passageway for air going into the lungs. It is also the organ of smell as the olfactory receptors are located in the nose. The inner lining of the nose is a ciliated mucous membrane with a rich supply of blood vessels. It has two functions:

1 To filter the air as it enters the system, trapping organisms and dust particles preventing their entry into the lungs.
2 To moisten and warm the air as it passes through.

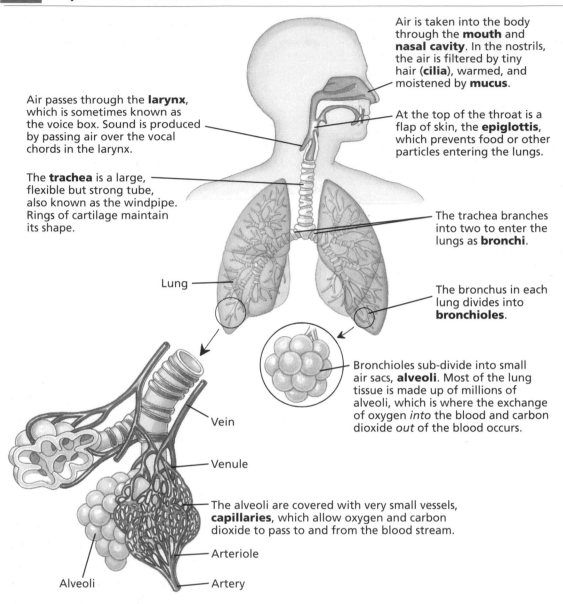

Air is taken into the body through the **mouth** and **nasal cavity**. In the nostrils, the air is filtered by tiny hair (**cilia**), warmed, and moistened by **mucus**.

Air passes through the **larynx**, which is sometimes known as the voice box. Sound is produced by passing air over the vocal chords in the larynx.

At the top of the throat is a flap of skin, the **epiglottis**, which prevents food or other particles entering the lungs.

The **trachea** is a large, flexible but strong tube, also known as the windpipe. Rings of cartilage maintain its shape.

The trachea branches into two to enter the lungs as **bronchi**.

Lung

The bronchus in each lung divides into **bronchioles**.

Bronchioles sub-divide into small air sacs, **alveoli**. Most of the lung tissue is made up of millions of alveoli, which is where the exchange of oxygen *into* the blood and carbon dioxide *out* of the blood occurs.

Vein

Venule

The alveoli are covered with very small vessels, **capillaries**, which allow oxygen and carbon dioxide to pass to and from the blood stream.

Arteriole

Alveoli

Artery

FIGURE NUMBER: 5.7 – The respiratory system.

The pharynx

Both the respiratory and digestive tracts share the pharynx as both air and food pass through this passageway. The tonsils are located here.

The larynx

This is the voice box which lies between the pharynx and the trachea. It is composed of cartilages and smooth muscle tissue. The larynx plays a part in respiration, speech and swallowing. Air passes through the larynx to the trachea; the passage of air over the vocal chords causes them to vibrate, producing sound. During the swallowing of food the larynx protects the airway as it is drawn up, shutting off the airway to prevent food entering.

The trachea

This is a tube about 4.5 inches long and 1 inch in diameter which extends from the larynx to the bronchi. It is composed of smooth muscle with C-shaped bands of cartilage at regular intervals along its length. These cartilagenous bands prevent the walls of the trachea from collapsing inwards. The function of the trachea is to maintain a permanently open pathway to the lungs. Any obstruction of this vital airway, even for a few minutes, will result in asphyxia (suffocation) and death.

The bronchi

The trachea eventually divides into two primary bronchi.

The right bronchus leads to the right lung.

The left bronchus leads to the left lung.

In structure, each bronchus is similar to the trachea, being composed of smooth muscle with C-shaped rings of cartilage at intervals along its length. As the bronchi enter the lungs they further subdivide into smaller secondary bronchi and then into even smaller bronchioles. The bronchioles further divide into minute tubes called alveolar ducts which terminate in sponge-like sacs called alveoli.

The lungs

The left and right lungs are cone-shaped organs which extend from their base on the diaphragm below, to their apex above the clavicles. They lie within the thoracic cavity protected by the ribs and the sternum. The left lung is composed of two lobes and the right lung is composed of three lobes. They are covered by the visceral pleura containing serous fluid which reduces friction and facilitates movement of the lungs during breathing. The lungs are composed of the tubes of the bronchial tree and the numerous sponge-like alveoli. The alveoli are surrounded by dense capillary networks. The function of the lungs is to provide a large surface area where the inspired air can come into close contact with the blood thus facilitating the rapid exchange of gases. This exchange takes place across the alveoli-pulmonary capillary interface. Oxygen, from inspired air, diffuses through the walls of the alveoli, through the walls of the surrounding capillary networks, into the blood to be transported around the body, to the tissue cells. Carbon dioxide from tissue cells is carried via the blood to the lungs. Here it diffuses through the capillary walls then in through the walls of the alveoli to be expired out of the lungs. This gaseous exchange is regulated by the partial pressure of the gases in the alveolar air and in the pulmonary blood. The gases diffuse across the gradient from high pressure to low pressure until equilibrium is reached. (Diffusion is the movement of molecules across a permeable membrane.)

Ventilation

Ventilation is the movement of air in and out of the lungs. As explained previously, ventilation is brought about by the contraction of the skeletal muscles which expand the thorax. The muscles involved are the diaphragm and the intercostal muscles which lie between the ribs. Ventilation is composed of two phases, *inspiration*, taking air into the lungs and *expiration*, expelling air out of the lungs.

During inspiration the external intercostal muscles contract, swinging the ribs outwards and upwards, rather like a bucket handle, and the sternum is pushed forward. This increases the thoracic cavity from side to side and from front to back. At the same time the diaphragm contracts to increase the cavity longitudinally. This increases the volume of the thorax and reduces the pressure within to below atmospheric pressure, consequently air rushes into the lungs. During normal expiration these muscles relax, the thoracic cavity returns to its normal size, the pressure increases to above atmospheric pressure and air rushes out. During forced respiration the internal intercostals contract pulling the ribs in and down, the diaphragm moves upwards, forcing air out.

Minute ventilation is the amount of air inspired (Vi) *or* expired (Ve) in one minute.

This will depend on how much air we breathe in per breath (at rest this is around 400–600 mL) and the number of breaths per minute (at rest 10–25 breaths/min).

Definitions of lung volume and capacities
- *Pulmonary ventilation* is the movement of air in and out of the lungs.
- *Tidal Volume* (Vt) is the volume of air inhaled *or* exhaled in one breath.
- *Minute ventilation* (VE) is the amount of air we exhale in one minute. At rest this is between 6–15 L/min but during maximal exercise this can increase to between 145–200 L/min. These increases are the result of an increase in the depth and rate of breathing.
- *Vital capacity* (VC) is the maximum volume forcefully expired after maximal inspiration.
- *Residual volume* (RV) is the volume remaining in the lung at the end of maximal expiration.
- *Total lung capacity* (TLC) is the volume of air in the lung at the end of maximal inspiration.

Respiratory response to exercise
- The respiratory and the cardiovascular systems closely interact to take in and transport oxygen to the contracting muscles and to remove carbon dioxide, a waste product of aerobic activity, from the muscles to the lungs. During exercise ventilation may be 15–30 times greater than at rest.
- When exercise commences there is a rapid rise in ventilation which may increase from a resting level of 6–15 L/min up to 145–200 L/min. This increase is possible because of: increased rate of breathing, and increased depth of breathing.

The initial rapid rise will tend to level off during steady state sub maximal exercise but will continue to rise during maximal effort.

- Improved strength and condition of the muscles of respiration.
- Improved elasticity and recoil property of lung tissue.
- Improved diffusion capacity across the alveolar–pulmonary capillary interface.
- An increase in the blood supply to and from the lungs.

Summary and aid to learning

The function of the respiratory system is the exchange of gases between the human body and the environment.

The system is composed of: the nose, pharynx, larynx, trachea, bronchi, bronchioles and the lungs made up of alveoli.

As air passes in through the nose it is warmed and filtered. It is further warmed as it passes through the pharynx and larynx.

The trachea divides into two primary bronchi: the right bronchus to the right lung and the left bronchus to the left lung.

The bronchi subdivide as they enter the lungs into smaller bronchi which further divide into brochioles. These end as small ducts which enter the alveoli.

There are two lungs containing the branches and alveoli.

How many lobes are there to each lung?

The inspired air must be brought into close contact with the blood for the exchange of gases to take place.

Study the text and state where the exchange takes place. Name the main gas that moves out of the lung into the blood and name the main gas that passes out of the blood into the lungs to be exhaled.

Ventilation is the movement of air in and out of the lungs. Inspiration is the taking of air into the lungs, in other words breathing in. Expiration is expelling air out of the lungs, i.e. breathing out.

The muscles of respiration contract to expand the chest during inspiration; they relax during expiration. Name the muscles of respiration.

Minute ventilation is the amount of air inspired or expired in one minute.

This will depend on the number of breaths per minute and the amount of air taken in per breath. Study the list of lung volume and capacities.

The respiratory system must work harder and faster during exercise to take in increased oxygen and to eliminate carbon dioxide.

Discuss the improvements that can be expected following a period of training.

QUESTIONS
1. Name the three main parts that make up the nervous system.
2. Give the function of each type of neurone.
3. Complete the following:
   a Axons carry impulses ... .
   b Dendrites carry impulses ... .
4. Name the chemical transmitter that transports an impulse across a synaptic gap.
5. Explain the function of proprioceptors.
6. Name the sensory receptor which relays information regarding the degree of stretch within a muscle.
7. Discuss the function of the cardio-vascular system during exercise.
8. Describe the pathway of oxygenated blood after it leaves the lungs.
9. Outline how the gases oxygen and carbon dioxide are transported in the blood.
10. Explain the term 'blood shunting' and outline why it occurs.
11. Explain the term venous return. How is it aided back to the heart.
12. Define the following:
    a Stroke volume
    b Heart rate
    c Cardiac output.
13. Explain how each of these is affected by exercise.
14. Discuss the effects on the heart of a period of long term training.
15. Explain the interaction between the cardio-vascular and respiratory systems during exercise.
16. Describe how oxygen passes from the external environment to the muscles.
17. Define the terms:
    a Tidal volume
    b Vital capacity
    c Total lung capacity.
18. Discuss how 'minute ventilation' increases from rest to maximal exercise and give values.
19. List the improvements found in the respiratory system following a period of training.

Chapter 6
Muscle work

Muscles work to produce or control movement at joints. When a muscle is working, tension force builds up within the muscle and the muscle may shorten, lengthen or remain the same length depending on the action required.

The muscle may be required to move a part, to control the effect of an external force or to hold a specific static position.

ISOTONIC, ISOMETRIC AND ISOKINETIC WORK

Muscle work or contraction is classified into isotonic and isometric and recently defined isokinetic.

Isotonic contraction – equal tone; as force is generated, the muscle changes in length throughout the movement but the tone remains the same. The muscle may shorten, when the work is known as *concentric work*, or the muscle may lengthen, when the work is known as *eccentric work*.

In practice it is not possible for the tone to remain the same throughout the full range of movement because of the difference in the angle of pull across the range. The degree of tension will vary with the position of the joint. For example, when performing a biceps curl with a weight in the hand, the tension developed will vary depending on the joint angle. The greatest tension is developed just before the angle of the elbow approaches a right angle. In fact, it has been shown that tension is maximal at 120 degrees; it decreases to the weakest point at 30 degrees. It follows that a muscle is only as strong as its weakest point which will limit the maximum weight that can be lifted. The muscle would only generate maximal tension at its weakest point, it will not be contracting maximally through the rest of the range. This is an obvious disadvantage to the athlete who requires strength throughout the range. Machines have now been developed to overcome this problem as explained below.

Isometric contraction – equal length; the length of the muscle does not change but there is an increase in tone. This is also known as static work.

Isokinetic contraction – equal speed; this is maximal contraction at constant speed throughout the range. Machines have been developed which adjust automatically to provide maximal resistance and constant speed throughout the range. This is of great benefit to athletes, as strength and speed gives power which is a major factor in peak performance. Although the lift will be a concentric contraction as in isotonic work, the tension will be maximal throughout the range.

LEARN
Isotonic – the muscle changes in length; in concentric contraction the muscle shortens; in eccentric contraction the muscle lengthens
Isometric or static work
No change in muscle length but there is an increase in tone
Isokinetic – maximal contraction at constant speed throughout the range.

Definitions and Examples

Isotonic work may be concentric or eccentric:

- Concentric work (isotonic shortening) – a muscle working concentrically shortens and thickens, the origin and insertion move towards each other and movement is produced in the joint.
  For example, in bending the elbow to lift a weight, the elbow flexors shorten to flex the elbow.
- Eccentric work (isotonic lengthening) – a muscle working eccentrically becomes longer and thinner as the origin and insertion move away from each other. The muscle pays out gradually to control the movement produced by some external force such as gravity, springs, etc.
  For example, when lowering a bucket of water to the ground, the elbow flexors lengthen and pay out gradually to lower the bucket smoothly downwards. If these muscles stopped working the bucket would drop rapidly due to the force of gravity.

Isometric work is also known as static work.

- A muscle working statically does not change in length, but there is an increase in muscle tone. The origin and insertion do not move and there is no joint movement.
  For example, when holding a bucket of water above the ground, the elbow flexors have to increase in tone to maintain the position, but there is no movement at the elbow joint.

Muscles can be made to work statically by pushing against immovable objects or by holding heavy weights or springs.

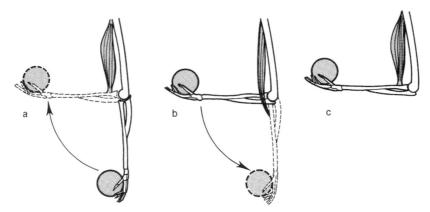

FIGURE NUMBER: 6.1 – (a) The biceps working concentrically to lift a ball.
(b) The biceps working eccentrically to lower a ball.
(c) The biceps working statically to hold a ball.

Isokinetic work (contraction against special isokinetic machines)
- The muscle contracts at constant speed and the tension developed within the muscle is maximum at all joint angles through full range. For example: straightening/extending the knee against the resistance applied by an isokinetic machine when the speed is kept constant – this tension generated in the quadriceps muscle will be maximal throughout the range.

Other examples of concentric, eccentric and static work

Concentric work

Another example of concentric work is standing and raising the arm to the side. This movement of abduction at the shoulder joint is brought about by the contraction of the deltoid. The deltoid becomes shorter and thicker as the insertion moves towards the origin, its power overcomes the pull of gravity and the arm is abducted. The deltoid is working concentrically.

Eccentric work

One way to lower the arm would be for all muscles to relax, so that gravity pulls the arm rapidly down to the side. In order to control this movement of adduction, the deltoid now 'pays out' with the insertion moving away from the origin so that the arm is lowered slowly in a controlled manner. The deltoid is working eccentrically.

Static work

To continue with the same example, the deltoid would work statically if the arm were held out in abduction, allowing no movement. Common static exercises are tightening and holding the gluteal muscles, the abdominals and the quadriceps.

Isokinetic work

The movement of the arms through the water during freestyle swimming.

The uses of muscle work

Concentric muscle work is the usual method used for muscle strengthening, although eccentric and static work should also be included. Maximal strength gains will not be achieved throughout the range.

Eccentric muscle work can sometimes be easier to perform and is useful when re-educating muscles if they cannot perform concentric work. Eccentric work in full and outer range (see below) maintains flexibility. Muscle soreness is greatest following eccentric contraction.

Static work is easy to perform, but muscle fatigue develops quickly. This is because the constant compression on the blood vessels and capillary networks impedes the blood flow, thus reducing the delivery of oxygen and nutrients and the removal of waste products.

Static work increases the blood pressure and should not therefore be performed by those with heart and blood pressure problems.

Static work should be practised for short periods, with frequent rest intervals. It is also important to perform static holding at different points throughout the muscle range.

Isokinetic work is the most effective work for strengthening muscles as maximal resistance is applied throughout the range which will result in equal improvement throughout the range. Muscle soreness is least following isokenetic contact.

TASK

Work with a partner.
While one of you performs a movement, the other should try to identify the type of muscle work, for example standing, swing the right leg out sideways. The abductors are working concentrically.

RANGE OF MOVEMENT

When muscles contract they move the joint through a certain range.

There are four ranges that a muscle or joint can work through:
1   *Full range* – from full stretch to full contraction, or vice versa.
2   *Outer range* – from full stretch to the mid-point of contraction, or vice versa.
3   *Inner range* – from the mid-point to full contraction, or vice versa.

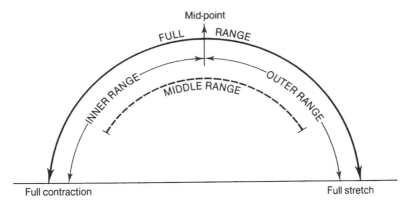

FIGURE NUMBER: 6.2 – The range of movement.

4 *Middle range* – any distance from the mid-point of the outer range to the mid-point of the inner range, or vice versa.

LEARN
There are four ranges of movement:
Full range   Inner range
Outer range   Middle range

Full range work is rarely used for normal activities, but it is essential for maintaining full joint mobility and muscle flexibility and is useful for reducing tension.

Outer-range work is difficult due to the angle of pull of the muscle, and energy is wasted in the compression of joint surfaces (shunting), but exercises in both the full and outer ranges prevent shortening of the muscles and maintain joint mobility. The outer range is used for stretching work.

Inner-range work is used when re-educating weak muscles and for strengthening work as the angle of pull is advantageous, but extreme inner-range work again wastes energy in pulling joint surfaces apart.

The middle range is the range in which muscles are most often used in everyday activities. They are more efficient in this range because the angle of pull of the muscle is nearer 90°, but full joint movement is never achieved in this range.

Remember:
■ inner- and middle-range work for re-educating weak muscles and strengthening exercises;
■ full-range work for mobilising joints and relieving tension;
■ outer-range work for stretching, preventing muscle shortening and maintaining flexibility and end of range movement at joints.

THE GROUP ACTION OF MUSCLES

LEARN

There are four different muscles or groups working when movement occurs. They are
- prime movers (agonists) – these produce the movement
- antagonists are the opposite group which relax
- synergists – these help the prime movers
- fixators – these fix or stabilise other joints

When muscles contract to produce movement, they work in groups. Each member of the group has a particular role to play, rather like the members of an orchestra. They work together in a synchronised manner to produce smooth, co-ordinated, efficient movement.

There are four different members, which are named according to their function. They are the agonists or prime movers, the antagonists, the synergists and the fixators:

- The *agonists* or *prime movers* are the muscles that contract to produce the required movement (prime action).

  For example, abduction of the hip joint is produced by the abductors; therefore the gluteus medius, the gluteus minimus and the tensor fasciae latae are the agonists or prime movers.

- The *antagonists* lie on the opposite side of the joint from the agonists. They are the opposite group, which must relax and lengthen in a controlled manner so that the movement produced by the agonists is performed smoothly.

  For example, when the abductors are contracting to abduct the hip the opposite group, the adductors, must relax. Therefore the adductors magnus, longus, brevis, pectineus and gracilis are the antagonists.

- The *synergists* assist the prime movers to produce the most efficient movement. They may alter the angle of pull of the prime mover or prevent unwanted movement.

  For example, during abduction of the hip the deep hip muscles will prevent the hip rotating, so that maximum effort is put into abduction. Therefore the piriformis and the obturator muscles are the synergists.

- The *fixators* ensure that the prime movers act from a fixed base. They stabilise and prevent unnecessary movements in surrounding joints.

  For example, during abduction of the hip joint the pelvis is held steady. Therefore the trunk side flexors and abductors of the opposite side are the fixators.

LEARN

Muscles acting on a joint are arranged around a joint. Those with opposite actions lie on opposite sides of the joint.
Flexors opposite extensors
Abductors opposite adductors
Medial rotators opposite lateral rotators

The agonists and antagonists are the most vital members of the group and require identification when analysing muscle work. When the agonists are contracting to produce movement, the antagonists must relax to allow the movement to take place. This is known as reciprocal relaxation and can be used as a technique for stretching muscles (see chapter 9). It is sufficient to remember that synergists and fixators are also contributing to the movement, as their identification is frequently difficult.

The muscles acting on a joint are arranged around the joint. Some are superficial while others are deep. The agonists and antagonists are arranged as opposite pairs – flexors opposite extensors, abductors opposite adductors, medial rotators opposite lateral rotators. When the flexors are the agonists, the extensors will be the antagonists and vice versa. Other smaller muscles will be the synergists and fixators. The patterns of movement are synchronised in the motor cortex and the appropriate impulses are conveyed to the muscles via their motor nerves.

The balance between agonists and antagonists is very important as tightness and shortening or over-stretching and weakness of one group will affect the function of the other. A muscle imbalance will be produced, resulting in stresses on the underlying joints and ligaments which may adversely affect performance. These stresses may also result in deformity and pain. Exercises must always be planned to maintain a balance between agonists and antagonists.

ANALYSIS OF MUSCLE WORK

All exercise schemes require careful planning to ensure that the set objectives are realised. For corrective schemes, the exercises must be carefully planned to target specific muscles or groups: some will require strengthening, while others will require stretching. For general schemes, all the main muscle groups must be included and balance maintained between opposing muscles.

Planning exercise schemes therefore requires the ability to analyse muscle work. First of all, the starting position must be considered, as this determines the effect of gravity on the movement. This is followed by identification of the moving joint, the direction of movement and the muscles producing that movement. Then we consider the type of muscle work and the range of movement.

To analyse muscle work follow this procedure:
1 Give the starting position.
2 Name the moving joint, e.g. hip, shoulder, etc.
3 Name the direction of movement, e.g. flexion, abduction, etc.
4 Name the prime movers, i.e. the muscles producing the movement.
5 Name the type of muscle work, i.e. concentric, eccentric or static.
6 Name the range of movement, i.e. inner, outer, middle or full.

The type of muscle work poses the most difficult problem to most students. Remember:
■   If the muscle is shortening and the origin and insertion are moving nearer to each other, the work is concentric.

- If the movement is produced by an external force such as gravity, weights or springs and the muscle is lengthening and paying out to control the movement, so that the origin and insertion are moving away from each other, the work is eccentric.
- If the muscle is contracting but producing no movement at the joint, the work is static.

LEARN

To work out which muscle or group is working, ask yourself the following questions:
What is the starting position?
Which joint is moving?
What is the direction of movement?
Which muscles are producing that movement?
Which type of muscle work is it?
(is the muscle shortening, lengthening or staying the same length)?
Which range is it moving through?

Exercises performed in different starting positions will have different muscle work, for example abduction and adduction of the hip joint performed in different positions, as shown below.

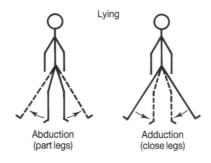

FIGURE NUMBER: 6.3a

Position:	lying supine
Movement:	part legs
Moving joint:	hip
Direction of movement:	abduction
Prime movers:	the abductors (gluteus medius, minimus and tensor fasciae latae)
Muscle work:	concentric (muscle shortens producing the movement)
Range:	inner
Movement:	close legs
Moving joint:	hip
Direction of movement:	adduction
Prime movers:	adductors (adductors longus, magnus, brevis, pectineus, gracilis)

Muscle work:	concentric
Range:	outer

When the legs are opened and closed in the lying position gravity does not affect the movement, since gravitational pull is downwards and this movement is in the horizontal plane.

Both the abductors and adductors work concentrically.

Side lying

Abduction
(leg raise)

Adduction
(leg lower)

FIGURE NUMBER: 6.3b

Now if we change the starting position but do the same movement the muscle work changes.

Position:	lying on side
Movement:	upper leg raise
Moving joint:	hip joint
Direction of movement:	abduction
Prime movers:	abductors (as before)
Muscle work:	concentric (muscle shortens)
Range:	inner

(This movement is against the pull of gravity.)

Movement:	lowering leg
Moving joint:	hip joint
Direction of movement:	adduction
Prime movers:	abductors (because gravity will pull the leg down)
Muscle work:	eccentric
Range:	inner

Gravity pulls the leg down, therefore the adductors do not need to work, but the abductors work eccentrically to prevent the leg from falling.

Thus in this starting position the muscle work changes: only the abductors work, first concentrically and then eccentrically to produce controlled movement and counteract the pull of gravity.

If we change the starting position yet again, the muscle work will change again.

Position:	lying with legs at right angles to trunk
Movement:	part legs

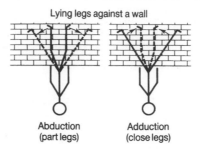

Lying legs against a wall

Abduction (part legs)   Adduction (close legs)

FIGURE NUMBER: 6.3c

Moving joint:	hip joint
Direction of movement:	abduction
Prime movers:	adductors (because gravity will pull the legs out)
Muscle work:	eccentric
Range:	outer

Movement:	close legs
Moving joint:	hip joint
Direction of movement:	adduction
Prime movers:	adductors
Muscle work:	concentric
Range:	outer

Only the adductors work in this position, first eccentrically to produce controlled movement and counteract the pull of gravity. They then work concentrically to draw the legs in.

TASK

Work out the muscle work of elbow flexion and extension in the following starting positions. (Remember that the biceps flexes the elbow and the triceps extends the elbow.)

a stride standing (arms at side) – raise hand to touch shoulder

b as above – lower hand back down

c yard stride standing – bring hand in to touch shoulder

d as above – bring hand back out to yard

e head rest stride standing – raise hand up to elevation

f as above – lower hand back to head.

THE CLASSIFICATION OF MOVEMENT

Movements may be classified as shown in Figure 6.4.

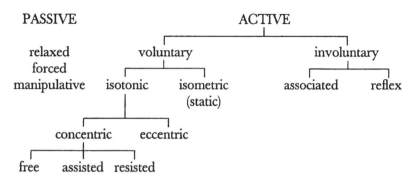

FIGURE NUMBER: 6.4

Passive movements

These movements are performed by an external force, and the client's own muscles are inactive, i.e. do not contract. The therapist moves the joint, but the client plays no active part. These movements are used to maintain or increase the mobility in joints.

They may be classified as:
- relaxed passive movements – performed within the existing range;
- forced passive movements – performed beyond the existing range;
- manipulative passive movements – these are forced movements performed under anaesthetic and are carried out to break down adhesions that are limiting joint movement.

Passive movements should be carried out under medical supervision only.

Active movements

These may be voluntary, i.e. under the control of the will, or involuntary, i.e. not under the control of the will.

Involuntary movements

These are not controlled by the will and may be:
- *reflex* movements, such as blinking or movement away from hot or painful conditions;
- *associated* movements, which are made by the fixators and synergists during active movements.

Voluntary movements

These movements are controlled by the will and are the result of the voluntary action of muscles. They may be:

- *isometric* (static), where the muscles do not change in length but increase in tone and no movement is produced at the joint;
- *isotonic*, where the muscles change in length and produce movement at the joints. Isotonic movements may be concentric (muscle shortening) or eccentric (muscle lengthening).

LEARN

Movement may be
- passive: these are performed by someone else or some extended force
- active: these are performed by the person's own muscles contracting

---

Concentric movements may be further subdivided into assisted, free and resisted:
- *Assisted active exercise* – when muscle power is inadequate to produce a desired movement, its power can be helped by the use of an external force acting with the muscle pull. The movement is thus assisted.
- *Free active exercise* is movement where the working muscles are subjected only to the forces of gravity acting upon the part being moved.
- *Resisted active exercise* is movement where the action of the muscles is resisted by an external force, e.g. weights, springs, etc. This resistance acts against the muscle pull. It can be increased progressively to develop muscle power and endurance.

Summary and aid to learning

There are three basic types of muscle contraction:

Isotonic, isometric and isokinetic.

Isotonic contraction can be subdivided into:

concentric contraction – when the muscle shortens, the origin and insertion come closer together.

eccentric contraction – when the muscle lengthens, the origin and insertion move away from each other, as the muscle pays out slowly to control any external forces acting on it.

Isometric contraction is also known as static contraction. The muscle develops tension but there is no change in length.

Isokinetic contraction – this is recently defined as maximum contraction at constant speed. Machines have been developed to keep the speed constant throughout the range. It has an advantage over isotonic contraction as strength gains will be equal throughout the entire range.

Work with a partner and perform concentric, eccentric and static contractions for different muscles in different starting positions.

When a muscle contracts it moves and moves the joint through a certain distance. This is known as 'the range of movement'. There are *four* ranges of movement: full, middle, inner and outer. If you think about these words they explain the range. Explain and demonstrate each range to a partner, using the biceps muscle.

Muscles must work as a group in order to perform smooth coordinated movement. The muscle which contracts to produce the movement is called the *prime mover* or *agonist*. The muscle on the other side of the joint, i.e. opposite the prime mover, must relax slowly to allow smooth movement to take place; this is called the *antagonist*. There are muscles that help the prime mover called *synergists*. Other muscles hold adjacent joints steady; these are called *fixators*.

When analysing muscle work you must give the *starting position* and identify:
- the *moving joint*
- the *direction* of movement, e.g. flexion, etc.
- the *prime mover*
- the *type* of muscle work, e.g. concentric, etc.
- the *range* of movement, e.g. middle, etc.

Practise this analysis with a partner; choose any movement and consider each of the above.

Passive movement is produced by some external force it requires no muscle contraction. Active movement is produced by muscle contraction.

QUESTIONS
1. Name the three main types of muscle work.
2. Define the terms *concentric work* and *eccentric work* and give one example of each.
3. Explain the four ranges of movement.
4. Name each member which contributes to the group action of muscles.
5. Define the terms:
    a prime mover (agonist)
    b antagonist.
6. List the points to consider when analysing muscle work.
7. Discuss the advantage of isokinetic contraction compared with isotonic contraction.
8. Analyse the muscle work of the following actions carried out in stride-standing position:
    a raise the arm out to the side to shoulder level
    b lower the arm back to the side.
    Now analyse these movements when the body is lying supine.
9. Define the terms *active movement* and *passive movement*.

Chapter 7
Physical principles relating to exercise

The science or study of body movement is known as kinesiology. As previously explained, movement is normally produced by muscles acting or pulling on bones, resulting in movement at joints. These movements are affected and governed by certain scientific principles. These need to be understood in order to identify muscle work and to devise effective and appropriate exercise schemes.

FORCE

A force is that which changes the state of rest or motion of an object. Any force acting on the body will make it move or affect its movement. When muscles contract they exert a force, which, if strong enough, will produce movement at the joint, for example the biceps muscle must contract with sufficient force to lift the forearm and bend the elbow. The power of the muscle must be great enough to overcome the resistance of any force pulling the other way, in other words the muscle force must be greater than the resisting force for movement to occur.

There are various external forces that can be used to resist movement, such as the pull of gravity or the use of weights, springs, pulley systems, multigyms, etc. Muscles are strengthened when they are made to work against progressively increasing forces.

Certain postural muscles are continually working against the force of gravity to maintain posture. If these muscles relaxed, the body would fall to the ground.

Gravity

This is the force that attracts or pulls everything towards the ground. It is a continual pull in a downward direction.

Gravitational pull affects most body movement and must be considered when planning exercises. Movements performed downwards (with gravity) will use different muscle work from those performed upwards (against gravity). Movements in the sagittal and frontal planes are affected by gravity, but movements in the horizontal plane are not.

Movements upwards, downwards or sideways will have different relationships with gravity and will require different muscle work. It is therefore very important to consider gravitational pull and to select appropriate starting positions when compiling exercise schemes (see chapter 8).

Anti-gravity muscles

The upright posture is maintained by particular muscle groups known as postural muscles or anti-gravity muscles. They must work continuously to oppose the pull of gravity and keep the body upright. Any weakness or imbalance of these muscles will affect body alignment and may result in postural deformities.

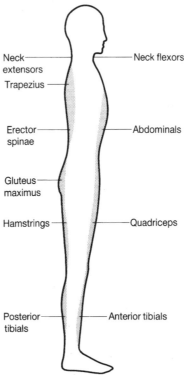

FIGURE NUMBER: 7.1 – Postural muscles.

Regular exercise will maintain muscle strength and balance, thus preventing abnormal postures. If deformities have developed, specific exercises must be practised to stretch the tight muscles and strengthen weak muscles.

The anti-gravity muscles are the anterior tibials, the posterior tibials, the quadriceps, the hip extensors (gluteus maximus and hamstrings), the erector spinae, the abdominals, the trapezius and the rhomboids, the neck extensors and the neck flexors.

The centre of gravity

This is an imaginary point at the centre of a body around which it is perfectly balanced. In the standing position the centre of gravity of the human body lies approximately at the second sacral vertebra, but this will vary with the shape and weight distribution of the individual. More weight on the top half raises the centre of gravity, whereas bending the knees or kneeling will lower it.

The lower the centre of gravity the more stable the object will be, so that a person in the lying position is more stable than a person in the standing position.

Stability is an important consideration when planning exercise, as the more stable the body is the easier it is to perform an exercise.

> **LEARN**
> The lower the centre of gravity, the greater the stability

The line of gravity

This is an imaginary line which falls perpendicularly (vertically) through the centre of gravity. When a person stands upright, the line of gravity passes through the vertex (top of the head), through the mid-cervical vertebrae, in front of the thoracic vertebrae, behind the bodies of the lumbar vertebrae, through the second sacral vertebra, slightly in front of the knee joint and in front of the ankle joint, ending between the ball of the foot and the heel.

The line of gravity is a useful measure when examining posture.

When the body adopts the correct posture, a line in the same plane but lateral to the line of gravity will fall through the lobe of the ear, the point of the shoulder (the acromion process), the hip joint, to the front of the knee joint (but behind the patella) and in front of the ankle joint, ending between the ball of the foot and the heel (see chapter 10). The line of gravity will not fall through all these points if posture is incorrect and will move as the position of the body changes.

Stability

The base of an object is that part that touches the ground. Any object with two or more feet on the ground will have a base that includes the area of the feet and the area of the space in between. The larger the area of the base the greater the stability.

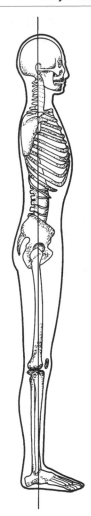

FIGURE NUMBER: 7.2 – The line of gravity.

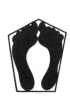 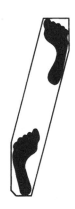 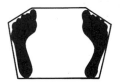

FIGURE NUMBER: 7.3 – The size of the base in standing, walk standing and stride standing.

When a person sits on a chair, the base includes the feet of the person and the area between the legs of the chair. When a person is lying down the area of the body surface on the ground is the base. This gives great stability, as it is a large base with a low centre of gravity.

LEARN
The larger the base the greater the stability

The stability of a body depends on the relationships between the centre of gravity and line of gravity and the base. As has already been mentioned, the lower the centre of gravity, the more stable the body will be. When the line of gravity falls near the centre of the base, the body is stable. As the line of gravity moves towards the edge of the base the body becomes increasingly unstable. If the line of gravity falls outside the base, the body falls over.

When the base is small it is difficult for the line of gravity to remain within it and the body easily falls over, but if the base becomes larger it is easier for the line of gravity to remain within it and the body is more stable. For example, if a person stands with the feet close together, the base is relatively small, being the area of the feet alone. Therefore, if the body moves forward, sideways or backward, the line of gravity will easily fall outside the base and the body will fall over.

However, if a person stands with the feet apart, as in stride standing, the base is much larger, being the area in between the feet as well as the area of the feet. The line of gravity will now stay within the base when the person leans over, and the body will not fall over as it is more stable. Arm and trunk movements are easier to perform when the body is more stable. Whenever the body moves into an unstable position, muscles are immediately brought into play to prevent the body falling over. The smaller the base and the higher the centre of gravity, the greater the muscle power and co-ordination needed to maintain the upright posture and the more difficult it will be to perform exercise. Other factors which increase stability are:

- increased body mass;
- friction between the feet and the ground;
- focusing the vision on a stationary object.

Newton's Laws of Motion

An understanding of these laws is useful when considering exercise, but in-depth study is not required.

Newton's laws state:
1 A body will continue in a state of rest or uniform motion in a straight line unless it is acted on by a force.
2 A change in acceleration of a body is directly proportional to the force and inversely proportional to the mass.
3 To every action there is an equal and opposite reaction.

The first law

The first law explains that a body will remain at rest or continue moving in a straight line unless it is affected by some force. The force may move a stationary object, or may make a moving object move faster or slower or may change the direction of movement. Forces can be applied singly, or many forces can work together in the same direction, or forces can work in opposition to each other.

We can look at examples in everyday life related to muscle work.

- A single force acting on an object will move it in the direction of that force. For example, a man pushing a car will move the car in the direction that he's pushing, providing he pushes hard enough. A muscle pulling on a bone will move the bone, providing the muscle pull is strong enough.
- If two or more forces are acting in the same direction the power or strength of the force will be the sum of the two forces. For example, two people pushing a car in the same direction will move the car in that direction. The strength of the force will be approximately the power of the first person plus the power of the second person and the work will be easier for each of them. In the same way, two muscles pulling together in the same direction will move a bone and the work will be easier for each muscle than if one was working alone.

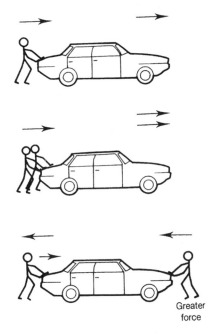

FIGURE NUMBER: 7.4 – The forces involved in pushing a car.

- Two forces acting in opposite directions will result in movement in the direction of the greater force. The strength of the force will be the difference between the two forces. For example, two people pushing a car in opposite directions will result in movement in the direction of the one pushing harder. Opposing muscles cannot contract together, because as the prime mover contracts the opposing antagonist always relaxes (this is controlled by nerve impulses and is known as reciprocal relaxation). However, muscles can be made to contract against external forces such as gravity, weights, springs, pulleys or machines. If the muscle force is greater than the external force, movement will occur in the direction of muscle pull. This principle is applied to improve muscle strength. A weight is selected that the muscle is just strong enough to lift, and this weight is lifted a set number of times. As the muscle responds and strengthens a greater weight is used and the procedure is repeated until the required strength is reached. If the muscle power and the weight are equal there will be equilibrium, and therefore no movement. If the weight is greater than the muscle power, movement will occur towards the weight. If the muscle is forced to lift too great a weight the myofibrils may tear, damaging the muscle.

The second law

The second law explains that an increase in speed will be directly proportional to the force, so that the greater the force, the greater the acceleration. It also depends on the mass: the greater the mass, the lower the acceleration.

For example, if two athletes of equal weight are pushing off from a starting block with equal force, they will accelerate at the same speed. However, if one is much heavier than the other he or she will accelerate more slowly, and will have to use greater force, i.e. muscle power, to produce the same acceleration.

The third law

The third law explains that every action has an equal and opposite reaction. This is important in ball games such as tennis and squash. The harder the ball is hit, the harder it hits the surface and the harder it rebounds. The surface applies a resistance force against the force of the striking ball. The resistance force from hard surfaces is greater than that from softer surfaces, which absorb some of the force. Hard court tennis is faster than grass court tennis, although the standard of play is equal. It is easier to run on hard surfaces than on soft surfaces, as there is a greater opposite reaction propelling one forward.

These opposing forces can cause problems for runners, as the constant jarring as the feet hit the ground may cause repetitive stress injuries such as shin splints and spinal problems.

When exercising it is an advantage to work on a sprung floor, which dissipates impact forces and reduces the risk of injury. Well-manufactured training footwear with cushioned soles should be worn to dissipate these forces.

(Some students may require other physical laws and principles related to speed, velocity and so on. These are not within the scope of this book and specialist texts should be referred to.)

Skeletal muscles produce the forces required for mobility. They start and stop movement, they maintain movement, they change the speed of movement, they may accelerate or decelerate actions and they change the direction of movement. Considerably more force is required to start and stop movement and to change direction than to maintain movement in the same direction.

LEVERS

Levers apply a force to produce movement about a point. Levers can be used to make work easier or harder. We are all familiar with the use of a lever to prise the lid off a tin of paint. When a coin is placed under the lid, and a force applied on the other side, the lid lifts up. If the coin does not work, we use a spoon handle or some longer rigid bar, and this will lift the lid because it has greater mechanical advantage. The principles of leverage also apply to body movement.

A lever is a rigid bar which moves around a fixed point called a fulcrum.

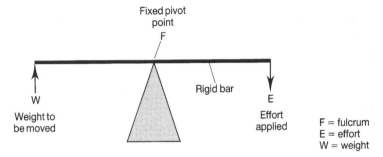

FIGURE NUMBER: 7.5 – A lever.

A force or effort (E) applied at one point on the lever moves a second force or weight (W) applied at another point.

The distance between the effort and the fulcrum is known as the effort arm (EA) and the distance from the weight to the fulcrum is known as the weight arm (WA).

A lever is balanced when
$$W \times WA = E \times EA$$
If the weight or length of the weight arm increases, the effort or length of the effort arm must also increase. Later we will see how this relates to increasing the work done by muscles.

In the body:
- the rigid bar is the bone;
- the fulcrum is the joint;
- the effort is the pull of the muscle at its point of insertion;
- the weight is the part being moved.

There are three different classes or orders of levers. They are different because of the position of the fulcrum in relation to the effort and the weight.

First order or class (EFW)

In the first order the fulcrum (F) lies between the effort (E) and the weight (W).

Here, the fulcrum may be nearer the weight, giving a longer effort arm, or may be nearer the effort, giving a longer weight arm. When the effort arm is longer than the weight arm there is mechanical advantage. If the weight arm is longer than the effort arm there is mechanical disadvantage.

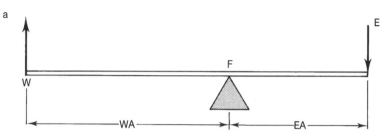

FIGURE NUMBER: 7.6a – The first order of levers.

We find examples of this first order in everyday life (e.g. a see-saw), but few in the body.

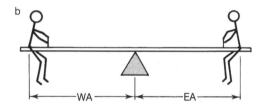

FIGURE NUMBER: 7.6b – Equilibrium on a see-saw.

If weight × weight arm = effort × effort arm, then the see-saw is balanced, but when one side is greater than the other the see-saw will move down at the end with the greater force. In the human body, during extension of the head the fulcrum lies at the cervical joints. The effort is supplied by the muscle pull at the point of insertion (upper fibres of trapezius) and the weight is the head being moved. In order to move the head backwards, the muscle power and the distance from the fulcrum must be greater than the weight of the head and its distance from the fulcrum.

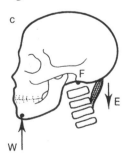

FIGURE NUMBER: 7.6c – Extension of the head.

Second order or class (FWE)

In this order the weight lies between the fulcrum and the effort.

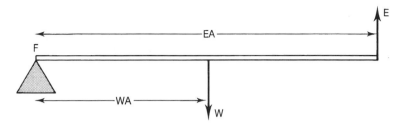

FIGURE NUMBER: 7.7a – The second order of lever.

Here, the effort arm will always be longer than the weight arm and consequently there will always be mechanical advantage. This is a lever of power.

A wheelbarrow has a fulcrum at the wheel, the weight in the middle and the effort at the handle. Because the effort arm is always longer than the weight arm, it is quite easy to lift a heavy load in a wheelbarrow.

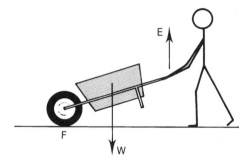

FIGURE NUMBER: 7.7b – Lifting a load in a wheelbarrow.

When raising the heel off the ground, the fulcrum is at the metatarso-phalangeal joints, the body weight falls down the leg to the ankle and the effort to lift the heel is from the plantar flexors (gastrocnemius and soleus) at their point of insertion.

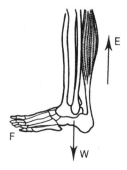

FIGURE NUMBER: 7.7c – Lifting the heel off the ground.

Third order of class (FEW)

In this order the effort lies between the fulcrum and the weight.

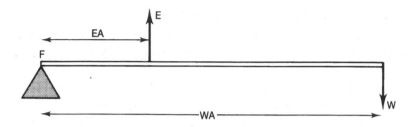

FIGURE NUMBER: 7.8a – The third order of lever.

Here the effort arm will always be shorter than the weight arm and therefore there will be mechanical disadvantage.

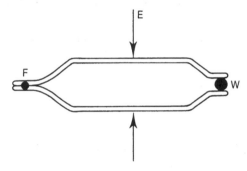

FIGURE NUMBER: 7.8b – A pair of sugar tongs.

A pair of tongs for picking up objects has the fulcrum at one end, the effort is applied in the middle and the weight lies at the other end.

During flexion of the elbow to lift the forearm, the fulcrum lies at the elbow joint. The effort is applied at the point of insertion of the biceps and brachialis muscles and the weight is the arm being lifted and any weight in the hand.

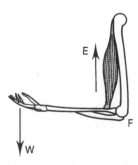

FIGURE NUMBER: 7.8c – Flexion of the elbow joint.

There is a larger number of third order levers in the body than any other. Although they are levers of mechanical disadvantage, they allow for speed and a wide range of movement.

Leverage related to muscle work

As explained previously, there are examples of all three types of lever to be found in the body, but there are far more of the third class, giving speed and a larger range of movement. When power is required we find the second class.

- The *fulcrum* is the joint where movement is taking place.
- The *effort* is provided by the muscle power exerted when the muscle contracts.
- The *effort arm* is the distance from the joint to the point where the muscle inserts (this cannot be changed).
- The *weight* is the part being moved, which can be increased by adding weight to the part.
- The *weight arm* is the distance from the fulcrum to the end of the moving part, which can be increased by adding length, such as a pole or dumb-bell.

Therefore we can increase the effort for the muscle by increasing the weight or lengthening the weight arm.

If muscle power (effort) × effort arm = weight × weight arm, everything is balanced and no movement will occur.

If we increase the muscle power so that muscle power (effort × effort arm) is greater than weight × weight arm, movement will occur.

If we then increase the weight or the length of the weight arm, greater muscle power will be required to produce movement.

This principle is used to strengthen muscles. The weight is progressively increased and the muscle is made to lift it a set number of times, with the result that the muscle become stronger (see chapter 9).

Examples

1   Increasing the work to strengthen abdominal muscles:
    Crook lying:
    - arms across chest, curl up (short weight arm)
    - hands on ears, curl up (longer weight arm)
    - arms stretched above head, curl up (longer weight arm)
    - arms across chest holding weight, curl up (increased weight)
    - arms stretched above head holding weight, curl up (increased weight arm and weight).
    This progression continues by increasing the weight to be lifted. Once the muscle can lift the weight 10 to 15 times, the weight can be increased.

2 Increasing the work to strengthen deltoid (Figure 7.9):
Stride standing:

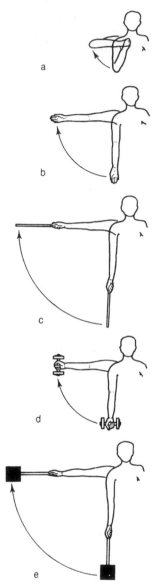

FIGURE NUMBER: 7.9 – Use of leverage to progress exercise.

- hand on shoulder, lift arm sideways (short weight arm)
- hand to side, lift arm sideways (longer weight arm)
- hand to side holding pole, lift arm sideways (longer weight arm)
- hand to side holding weight, lift arm sideways (increased weight). This weight can be increased as the muscle gets stronger
- hand to side holding weight at the end of the pole, lift arm sideways (longer weight arm and increased weight).

> **TASK**
> Show progression for the abductors of the hip joint in the side-lying position using the above five steps.

Summary

A *force* is that which changes the state of rest or motion of an object.

When a muscle contracts it exerts a pulling force on the bone of attachment, making it move.

Gravity is the force which pulls everything towards the ground.

Anti-gravity muscles are the muscles which contract to keep us upright. They work against the force of gravity; if they relaxed the body would fall to the ground.

Centre of gravity refers to the point at the centre of an object around which it is perfectly balanced.

The centre of gravity of the human body, in the standing position, is around the second sacral vertebra but this will vary with weight distribution. The lower the centre of gravity the more stable the object.

The *line of gravity* falls perpendicularly through the centre of gravity.

The base of an object is that part that touches the ground; the larger the base the more stable the object.

Explain how the base and the centre of gravity of an object affects its stability.

Levers apply a force to produce movement about a point.

A *lever* is a rigid bar which moves around a fixed point called a fulcrum. A force or effort is applied at one point to move a second force or weight applied at another point.

List the parts of a lever related to body parts and movement.

There are *three* types/orders of levers which are different because of the position of the fulcrum in relation to the effort and weight.

Draw a diagram of each type of lever and give an example of where each is to be found in the body.

We can increase the effort for a muscle, that is make it work harder, by increasing the weight or lengthening the weight arm.

There are more type three levers in the body than any other. These are levers of speed.

QUESTIONS

1. Define the terms *gravity* and *centre of gravity*.
2. Where is the approximate position of the centre of gravity in the human body?
3. When assessing posture, list the points through which the line of gravity will fall.
4. Complete the following:
   The base of an object is that part which … .
5. Give any three factors which influence the stability of a body.
6. Explain why it is preferable to exercise on a sprung floor.
7. Draw diagrams to illustrate the three classes of levers.
8. Relate the parts of a lever to the human body.
9. Give two ways in which leverage can be used to increase the resistance to muscle work.
10. Show two ways of using leverage to make the following exercise harder for the gluteus maximus:
    prone lying, raise the leg off the floor, knee bent to right angle.

Chapter 8
Starting positions

When writing out exercise schemes it is vital to state the starting position. This is easily done if schemes are written in two columns: one for the starting position, the other giving instructions for the exercise. The age and agility of the client will influence the choice of the starting position. The older or less agile client may well require a more stable starting position.

There are five basic starting positions:
- Lying (also known as supine lying)
- Kneeling
- Sitting
- Standing
- Hanging.

These basic positions can be modified to increase or reduce the difficulty of the exercise.

Modifications are made to:
- raise or lower the centre of gravity;
- increase or decrease the size of the base to change stability;
- increase or decrease leverage;
- provide adequate fixation of the body so that specific movements can be performed with maximum concentration;
- increase or decrease the muscle work required to maintain the position;
- ensure maximum support for relaxation.

Modifications of starting positions

■ Lying: prone lying, side lying, half lying, crook lying, crook lying with pelvis lifted.

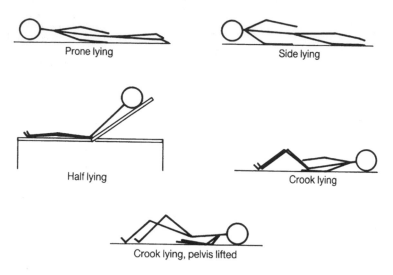

FIGURE NUMBER: 8.1 – Modifications of lying.

■ Kneeling: prone kneeling, inclined prone kneeling, heel sitting, half kneeling.

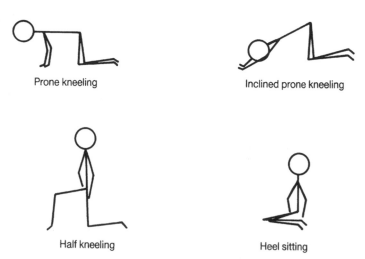

FIGURE NUMBER: 8.2 – Modifications of kneeling.

■ Sitting: crook sitting, long sitting, astride sitting, side sitting, stoop sitting, fall out sitting.

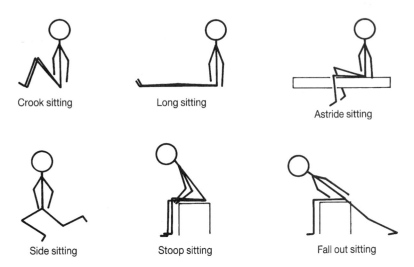

FIGURE NUMBER: 8.3 – Modifications of sitting.

■ Standing: toe standing, stride standing, walk standing, step standing, lax stoop standing, stoop standing.

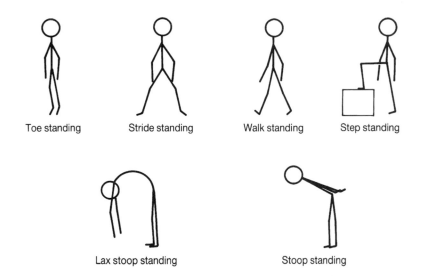

FIGURE NUMBER: 8.4 – Modifications of standing.

■ Hanging: stride hanging, knee bend hanging.

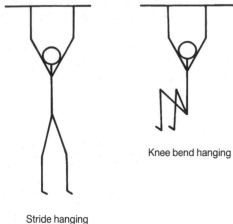

Knee bend hanging

Stride hanging

FIGURE NUMBER: 8.5 – Modifications of hanging.

The position of the arms is also very important and this is usually written first, e.g. bend stride standing.

■ Arm positions: wing, low wing, across bend, under bend, bend, reach, yard, stretch, head rest.

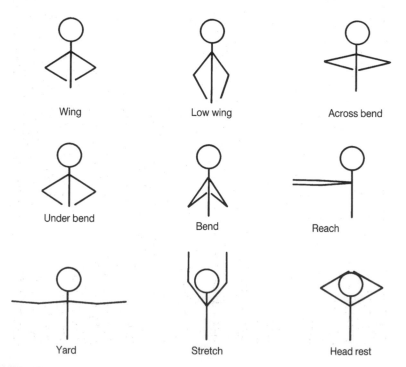

Wing

Low wing

Across bend

Under bend

Bend

Reach

Yard

Stretch

Head rest

FIGURE NUMBER: 8.6 – Arm positions.

PART B
Training for Fitness

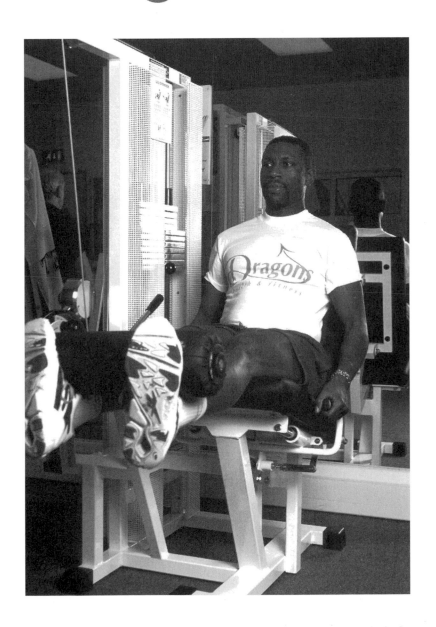

Introduction

Fitness may be defined as having sufficient energy and skill to cope in one's environment. Fitness is specific to the individual and ranges from the optimum fitness required by top athletes through to the lowest level required barely to cope with daily tasks.

Fitness and health are interrelated, but it is important to distinguish between the two. Health may be defined as 'freedom from disease' or 'a state of physical, mental and social well-being'; it is therefore possible to be healthy (free from disease) but unfit. It is also possible to be superbly fit and compete at the highest level while suffering ill health. Many top athletes continue competing or training when suffering from colds, infections, and so on.

Improving fitness means improving the physiological functioning of the various body systems, which in turn will improve one's capacity to function, resulting in an improved quality of life. Improvement is gained by overloading the systems, in other words by making demands on them over and above those required by normal activities, and continuing progressively to work them harder.

Chapter 9
The components of fitness

Before we can begin to improve fitness levels we must understand all the components that contribute to overall fitness. They can be defined in the following way:

Cardio-respiratory endurance means improving the condition of the heart and lungs, thus improving the delivery of nutrients and oxygen to the tissue cells.

Muscle strength means improving muscle maximum strength which will make activities easier.

Muscle endurance means improving the ability of muscles to contract for longer periods.

Flexibility means improving the suppleness of connective tissue components within the muscles which will improve extensibility and elasticity. It also improves the tensile strength and extensibility of ligaments and tendons. These factors will enable the tissues to withstand excessive forces, reducing the likelihood of injury.

Skill refers to accurate performance with little or no waste of energy. It is largely a function of the nervous system which initiates, controls and co-ordinates all activities.

Speed refers to the distance moved in a specific time. Some activities will require fast speed while others require slow control. Speed is an important factor in most sport because improved speed and strength will result in greater power.

Body composition refers to the ratio of body fat and fat-free tissue. It is dependent on energy balance which is the balance between energy consumed (the food eaten – calories in) and energy expended, (the amount of activity undertaken – calories out).

Nutrition refers to the foods we eat and the role they play in sustaining life. Good nutrition means eating the required amount of a variety of foods which will enable the body to function at maximum efficiency.

Rest and relaxation means allowing the body sufficient time to recover following activity. The more intense the activity the longer the rest period should be. Many physiological improvements continue into the rest period. Adequate rest will prevent chronic fatigue.

Relaxation means freedom from stress and is related to rest and anxiety states. Stress adversly affects the function of many body systems. Consequently reducing stress factors will enable the body to function more efficiently.

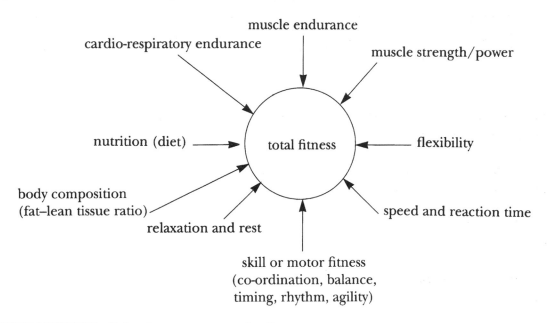

FIGURE NUMBER: 9.1 – Input necessary for fitness.

When we consider the concept of improving fitness it becomes obvious that this means different things to different people. Fitness is specific to the individual and the required improvement depends on the current level of fitness and desired fitness outcome. For an elderly person an improvement may be achieved simply through improved nutrition and a low level of increased strength and flexibility, while the peak performing athlete will require maximum levels of fitness in those systems related to his/her activity. Therefore a training programme must target the components where improvement is required. The weight lifter will require the maximum possible strength, the sprinter will require strength in the 'push off the block' muscles and anaerobic capacity; the marathon runner will require aerobic capacity; the ballet dancer will require flexibility, strength and aerobic capacity. Most sports will require a combination of many components and it is important to guard against overdevelopment of one at the expense of another. The most important questions to consider before embarking on a training programme are:

What is the current level of fitness?

What is the desired outcome or goal?

Planning

There are several important principles to consider when planning or embarking on any training programme.

Specificity

This means that the exercise/training routine must be specific to those muscles or energy systems targeted for conditioning, i.e. those used in the sport or performance. This is because training effects are generally not transferable; strength training will not improve cardio-vascular endurance or vice versa.

Overload

This means that the appropriate systems are stressed beyond normal requirements. Overload must always be appropriate to the fitness level of the individual; too little will not produce any improvement, too much can cause damage. Overload may be adjusted by increasing or decreasing one or all of the following:
- intensity: the degree of stress applied; it should be sufficient to produce some discomfort
- frequency: the frequency of the training sessions; the number of sessions per week;
- duration: the length of time of the exercise session or programme.

Progression

This means that the exercises/overload must become progressively harder for improvement and adaptation to be achieved. Progression must be steady and gradual.

Training threshold

This refers to the minimum intensity of exercise required to bring about improvement, e.g. to improve cardio-vascular endurance an individual must exercise at 60–80 percent of maximum heart rate (MHR) for 20–30 minutes, three times per week. 60 percent indicates the minimum intensity, this must be increased progressively as fitness develops. The very fit can work 90 percent MHR.

Reversibility

This refers to the loss of training effect if an individual stops exercising or if the intensity of training decreases. Training effect will regress within just two weeks and there will be considerable loss of fitness after a period of four to six weeks after training stops. The effects of short duration training regress more quickly than the effects of long duration training.

CARDIO-RESPIRATORY ENDURANCE

(Cardio-vascular, cardio-pulmonary and aerobic endurance are all terms used for this aspect of fitness). They all refer to the efficiency of the heart, circulation and lungs to take in, transport and transfer oxygen to muscle tissue.

Before exercise begins, the body is in a balanced state known as homeostasis, where the systems meet the body's metabolic needs. When exercise begins, the systems must respond rapidly to the increased demand for nutrients and particularly oxygen to produce ATP. If the demand (overload) is regularly and progressively increased the systems will respond and their physiological functioning will improve. The capacity of the body to work aerobically will increase, i.e. to utilise the aerobic energy system.

> **LEARN**
> Endurance training involves low intensity work over a period of time. It trains the body to provide and utilise oxygen, thus increasing aerobic capacity

Cardio-respiratory endurance improves as a result of low intensity, long duration training, which will improve the capacity to utilise the aerobic energy system. If the activity becomes too fast and vigorous, the systems will be unable to supply oxygen fast enough to meet the demand and the work will become anaerobic and endurance will not improve. Short bursts of fast activity will improve the capacity to utilise the anaerobic systems, i.e. ATP – PC system and the lactic acid system.

Training methods to improve cardio-respiratory endurance (aerobic capacity)

Cardio-respiratory endurance will improve in response to regular long duration, low intensity aerobic activities such as:

- jogging/running
- swimming;
- walking;
- treadmill running
- cross-country skiing;
- any aerobic dance or exercise programmes.

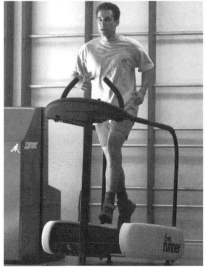

FIGURE NUMBER: 9.2

In order to maintain a training effect and improve fitness the work load must be gradually and slowly increased. As previously explained the three variables to consider are:

■ the intensity of the exercise – how hard it is;
■ the frequency of exercise – how often it is performed;
■ the duration of exercise – how long the programme lasts.

Intensity

Heart rate increases with exercise, therefore it is an excellent indicator of how hard the body is working. The heart rate varies considerably between different people and in the same person under different conditions. The heart rate is the same as the pulse rate and can be taken at pulse points throughout the body. The usual point for reading pulse rate is at the wrist (the radial pulse point). Participants in any training programme must be taught to take his/her pulse rate (see Chapter 14).

> ### LEARN
> The heart rate indicates the intensity at which a person is exercising

■ The average male resting pulse is between 72–76 beats per minute.
■ The average female resting pulse is between 76–80 beats per minute.

These are average values and considerable variations will be found. Fit people have a far lower resting pulse rate than the unfit. Endurance athletes may have pulse rates as low as 30–40 beats per minute.

> ### LEARN
> A person's maximum heart rate is the maximum rate at which it is safe to exercise.
>   An unfit person should not exceed 60 percent of maximum heart rate but should increase gradually up to 85–90 percent as fitness improves.

Maximum heart rate

To obtain an estimate of maximum heart rate (MHR) deduct the client's age from 220. For example, for a 40-year-old, maximum heart rate will be $220 - 40 = 180$ beats per minute.

> ### LEARN
> To calculate a person's maximum heart rate deduct his/her age from 220

The pulse rate must not exceed this MHR during aerobic exercise as it will produce too much stress. Healthy adults should exercise at a target heart rate of 60–90 per cent of their maximal heart rate depending on their current level of fitness. Those who are unfit should exercise at the lower end while those who are already quite fit should exercise at the higher end of their maximum range. Initially effort should be 60 per cent of MHR. For a 40-year-old this will be:

$$180 \times \frac{60}{100} = 108 \text{ beats/min. (this is the target heart rate or training rate)}$$

> **LEARN**
>
> The target heart rate is the rate at which the person should be exercising. It will be a percentage of maximum heart rate (60–90 percent).
>
> | Beginners | Intermediate | Advanced |
> |-----------|--------------|----------|
> | 60–70% | 70–80% | 80–90% |
>
> These will increase as fitness develops

The client should exercise with sufficient intensity to maintain this pulse rate for 15–30 minutes' duration two to three times per week. After four to six weeks it will be safe to exercise at 70 per cent of maximum heart rate providing there have been no problems.

$$180 \times \frac{70}{100} = 126 \text{ beats/min.}$$

Eventually, this will build up to 80–85 per cent even 90 per cent of MHR

Therefore, for this client

Age	MHR	Target Zone
40	180	108–161

> **LEARN**
>
> To maintain or increase levels of fitness any one or any combination of the following must increase: intensity, duration, frequency

Duration

This is the actual time that a person is exercising at the target heart rate. It does not include the warm-up and cool-down periods. This part of an exercise programme will last for 15–30 minutes. Initially, after a warm-up and stretch of 15–20 minutes, the client will perform a 15-minute programme, maintaining the target heart rate, and then cool down. This time will gradually increase to 30 minutes as fitness improves.

Duration is also used to describe the length of the training programme, e.g. 12–16 weeks.

Frequency

This is the number of sessions per week, which may be two to three times a week for an unfit beginner, moving up to three to four times per week as fitness improves. Athletes who compete in endurance, activities train for 4–5 days/week or more.

Selecting the training programme

The programme must be selected to meet the needs of the individual and to target the energy systems where improvement is required. Various forms of running can be selected to target the different energy systems; the intensity and duration will determine which energy system will 'kick in'. All running will commence with the ATP–PC system but as previously stated, a programme consisting of low intensity, long duration, steady state activities will utilise the aerobic system. Training will increase the capacity of this aerobic energy system and improve the physiological functioning of the heart and lungs. High intensity, short duration, fast activities will utilise and improve the anaerobic energy systems. Most sport and general fitness routines will utilise the three energy systems at some point or another depending on the availability of oxygen which depends on the intensity of the activity. The following suggested training methods can be manipulated to suit the requirements of the individual. Detailed training routines are not within the scope of this book.

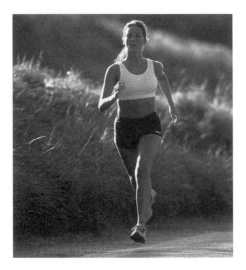

FIGURE NUMBER: 9.3

To train the aerobic system/endurance training

■ *Jogging* involves low level effort over a long period of time. Jogging for 3–6 miles at a very slow pace at 60–80 per cent of maximal heart rate.

■ *Long continuous running or slow distance running* involves low level effort over a long period of time. Running 3–5 miles at a steady slow pace but slightly faster than jogging. Beginning at 60 per cent of maximal heart rate, increasing to 85–90 per cent as fitness develops.

■ *Continuous fast running* involves running 1–2 miles at a steady fast pace, at approximately six minute mile pace. The distance has now been reduced but the pace has increased.

To train aerobic and anaerobic energy systems

1 Varied pace running
2 Interval training

3 Pick up sprint training

◼ *Varied-pace running* (Swedish Fartlek). This varies the pace at specific intervals through-out the run. Continuous steady-pace running is interrupted at intervals by quick sprints. This will combine both anaerobic and aerobic energy systems and is a more realistic training for most sports. It can be varied to use only aerobic systems if low effort is used in all stages.

It may involve running over different terrain, through forests and fields, uphill and downhill, on sand, gravel and grass.

Tracks are very carefully graded for their degree of difficulty. A programme may include:

1 10–15 minutes' jogging;
2 five minutes' rapid walk;
3 one mile slow distance running;
4 ten minutes' rapid walk;
5 five sprints interspersed with jogging over 100 metres.

◼ *Interval training*. This involves fast training interspersed with slow work, performed in a certain amount of time or over a measured distance. The slow or light work period allows the oxygen debt incurred during the fast work to be repaid. This method will improve both aerobic and anaerobic systems.

◼ *Pick-up sprint training*. This increases the speed of work. It begins with walking, moving on to jogging, then striding and sprinting, and ending up with walking again. The process is repeated as often as possible. This improves both aerobic and anaerobic systems and trains athletes to pick up speed quickly.

To train the anaerobic systems

◼ *Sprint training* involves repeated sprints of 60–70 yards with complete recovery in between.

◼ *Hollow sprints* involves sprinting interrupted by a recovery period of jogging or walking, e.g. sprint 60 yards, jog 60 yards, walk 60 yards, repeat until fatigued.

◼ *Cross-training*. Many athletes believe in and derive benefit from cross-training. This combines different forms of training. For example, cycling may be combined with swimming: the swimming will not improve cycling prowess, but it will maintain endurance qualities while allowing the recovery of the cycling muscles. It is also more interesting and motivating to add variety rather than keep to one training mode.

The effects of endurance training

Immediate Response

◼ The heart rate increases from around 80 to 180 beats per minute.
◼ The heart pumps out a larger volume of blood per beat (stroke volume).
◼ An increase in cardiac output which is stroke volume × heart rate from around 6 L/minute at rest to 30 L/minute during exercise.

- The flow of blood to the contracting muscles is greatly increased as blood is shunted from other organs such as the stomach.
- The rate and depth of ventilation increases. During exercise the volume of air breathed in and out of the lungs may be 30 times greater than that breathed in at rest.

After a period of training there will be further effects

- The heart increases in size and volume.
- The efficiency of the heart improves: it pumps out a larger volume of blood per beat (stroke volume) and therefore a larger quantity per minute (known as cardiac output).
- The heart rate decreases: the heart rests for a longer period, which reduces the workload on the heart. Endurance athletes may have heart rates as low as 40 beats per minute.
- There is an increase in the size and number of blood vessels in the heart and skeletal muscle.
- There is an increase in the size and density of capillary networks, supplying blood to the heart and skeletal muscle, with improvement in the delivery of oxygen and the removal of waste.
- There is an increase in the haemoglobin content of the blood which increases its oxygen carrying capacity.
- There is an increase in the size and number of mitochondria, which enables oxygen to be used more efficiently.
- There is an increase in glycogen stores and glycolytic enzymes.
- The aerobic capacity (VO_2max) is increased.
- The anaerobic threshold is raised, so that aerobic metabolism is used for longer periods, increasing the capacity to exercise without fatigue.
- The rate and depth of respiration increases, improving ventilation.
- Fats are utilised for energy production, which reduces body fat.
- Bones are strengthened in response to the stresses placed on them.

Dangers of Endurance Training

- Repetitive stress injuries, mainly of the ankles, knees and back, and shin splint injuries.
- Dehydration.

Precautions

- Perform adequate warm-up.
- Build up the training gradually. Do not exceed maximum heart rate (MHR). Begin at 60 per cent of MHR, working up to 80–90 per cent as fitness develops.
- Do not exercise if there is any pain present in musculoskeletal structures.
- Do not exercise if suffering from colds, fevers, flu, etc.
- Stop exercising if pain develops.
- Drink fluid after the training session or during long-distance running to prevent dehydration.
- Wear well-fitting, well-cushioned, appropriate footwear.
- Wear loose, absorbent clothing.
- Perform adequate cool-down.

Improving muscle fitness

Muscle response to overload training will differ, depending on the type of training:

- Muscle strength will increase in response to progressive overload over a period of time. Strength develops through high resistance with low repetitions.
- Muscle bulk will increase with strength, but one or two lifts at maximal resistance must be performed to improve bulking.
- Muscle endurance will increase in response to low resistance with high repetitions.
- Muscle power and explosive power will increase in response to plyometric training, involving muscle contraction following a rapid stretch.

> **LEARN**
>
> In response to progressive overload, muscles respond and improve. Muscles become stronger and bigger. Muscle power and explosive power will also improve

Muscle strength

This refers to the maximal force a muscle can develop against resistance. It is measured by the maximum weight that can be lifted in a single effort. This is known as one repetition maximum (1 RM). It is established by trial and error, using increasingly heavy weights, until the maximum is reached, for example by performing one lift of 10 kg, one of 12 kg and one at 14 kg, etc., until the maximum weight that can be lifted is reached.

Overloading a muscle with a weight of over two-thirds of the muscle's maximum load over a period of time will increase strength and bulk.

Initially, an increase in strength is the result of the recruitment of more motor units. Each motor unit stimulates a large number of muscle fibres to contract. Therefore, the more motor units recruited, the more fibres will be contracting, which will increase strength. Further strength develops as a result of an increase in the contractile proteins (myosin and actin) and in the size and number of myofibrils. These factors also increase muscle bulk.

Muscles will strengthen if they are made to contract against progressively increasing resistance.

> **LEARN**
>
> Muscle strength is the maximal force a muscle can develop against resistance

Resistance may be applied in many ways, but some of these methods are not measurable, and so accurate progression is not possible. Muscles can be made to work against:

- one's own body weight, e.g. press-ups – not measurable;
- the resistance provided by a partner, e.g. pushing or pulling against a partner – not measurable;
- water – not measurable;

- specialised equipment, such as rowing machines, exercise bikes, multigyms;
- free weights, e.g. sand bags, weight boots, ankle and wrist weights, dumb-bells and bar bells;
- springs and pulleys;
- weight machines are now very sophisticated and technologically advanced and can be found in gyms and fitness centres. They are the most popular method of weight training for athletes and fitness enthusiasts.

LEARN

Resistance may be applied to

Isotonic contraction $\begin{cases} \text{eccentric} \\ \text{concentric} \end{cases}$

Isometric contraction
Isokinetic contraction

Strength training programmes

Programmes may be required to improve overall body strength or to target specific muscles or groups related to sport or athletic performance. The following principles apply to any strength training programme.

Weight Training Principles

Overload

Muscles must be overloaded to gain strength; resistance must exceed that normally encountered. The resistance should be 66 percent of 1 (RM) repetition maximum or over. This is the minimum overload that will achieve a strength gain. If a muscle is underloaded, the present level of strength will be maintained but will not increase.

Progression

The overload must be progressive, it must increase as strength develops. As soon as the muscle can perform 2–4 extra lifts without fatigue, the load must be increased.

Arrangement of exercise

The routines should be organised so that succesive exercises do not involve the same muscle or group of muscles. The routine must be planned to include different areas consecutively, i.e. thigh, chest, lower back, buttocks, calf, shoulders and upper back, abdomen, upper arms. This ensures that muscles have an adequate time to recover, preventing fatigue.

Specificity

If strength is required for a specific sport or activity, the programme should be planned so that the muscles used in that sport or activity are exercised. If possible the exercise should simulate the normal pattern of movement used in the sport to reinforce the pattern of movement in the brain.

Recovery
Time should be allowed for recovery both between sets of lifts and between training days. Training three times per week will allow adequate rest time but still achieve strength gains.

Planning strength programmes
Muscle strengthening, otherwise known as weight training, usually involves concentric contractions against resistance. However, as discussed in chapter 6 there are three other types of contraction, namely eccentric, isometric and isokinetic contractions which can also be used.

Weight training programmes can be designed for each type of contraction as outlined below.

ISOTONIC strength training programmes
These exercises are dynamic and involve concentric muscle shortening and/or eccentric muscle lengthening, which will result in joint movement.

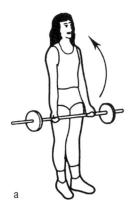
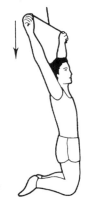

a   b

THE PYRAMID METHOD

FIGURE NUMBER: 9.5 – (a) Weight training for biceps.
(b) Weight training for latissimus dorsi.

Contraction is usually performed against weights, barbels or weight machines and uses the repetition maximum (RM) principle.

As the muscle contracts to lift the weight, the resistance is applied to concentric work. This is referred to as the positive phase and is the more effective phase for increasing strength and bulk.

Resistance is applied to eccentric work as the part is lowered back to the starting position. This is referred to as the negative phase.

The weight selected will depend on strength but must be over 66 percent of 1 RM.

As previously explained, repetition maximum is the maximum load that a muscle or group of muscles can lift a set number of times.

One repetition maximum (1 RM) is the maximum load that a muscle or group can lift only once before fatigue. Six repetition maximum (6 RM) is the maximum load that a muscle or group can lift six times before fatigue.

The contractions are organised into sets. One to five sets are repeated with a short pause between each set. Each set will consist of a certain number of contractions known as repetitions. A typical programme might be:

1 to 5 sets, of 6 to 10 contractions, 3–5 times per week for 6–10 weeks.

These factors can be manipulated to suit the individual and will depend on the rate at which strength gains have been achieved. Adequate rest is essential both between sets and between sessions to avoid chronic fatigue.

It is possible to use heavier loads for eccentric work thus gaining extra strength and bulk. This is favoured by very experienced lifters as part of their routine. The technique involves using two assistants to lift a heavy load into position (slightly too heavy for the concentric phase), which is then lowered slowly by the lifter.

Recording data

It is very important to record accurate details of the programme and progress. Measurements of bulk and strength taken at regular intervals under the same conditions will indicate progress. These measurements must be recorded before commencing the programme, and then every four weeks. Firstly:

- measure bulk with a tape measure placed around the widest point; always measure at the same point; record
- measure strength by the maximum weight which can be lifted in a single lift (1 RM); record 1 RM

During each session, the following data must be recorded:

- the load (the weight that is lifted)
- the repetitions (the number of times the weight is lifted without a rest – it is usual to select 6–10 lifts)
- the number of sets performed. Select 1–5 sets and allow 1 minute rest period between each set. These are recorded as follows:

    10 kg × 8 reps × 3 sets

As strength develops, the weight or number of sets is increased.

For improving strength, 'heavy load low repetitions' is the format: the weight lifted should be at least two-thirds of the maximum possible weight – over 66 percent of 1 RM. Beginners should practise initially with low weights until they have perfected the technique.

It is possible to vary the routines; the following are examples of effective but simple systems.

EXAMPLE 1

Establish 1 RM and calculate 80 percent of this, which will be the starting weight. If 1 RM = 25 kg, the weight will be 20 kg. This would be lifted 6–8 times and recorded as:

$$20 \text{ kg} \times 8 \times 1$$
$$20 \text{ kg} \times 8 \times 2$$
$$20 \text{ kg} \times 8 \times 3$$

EXAMPLE 2

Establish 10 RM (the weight that can be lifted 10 times). The first set of 10 lifts is performed with 50 percent of this weight, the second set with 75 percent and the third set with 100 percent. If 10 RM was 20 kg, this would be recorded as:

$$10 \text{ kg} \times 10 \times 1$$
$$15 \text{ kg} \times 10 \times 2$$
$$20 \text{ kg} \times 10 \times 3$$

The weight is increased as strength develops. The repetitions and sets may also be increased, but increasing the weight is the most essential.

Allow 48 hours between training sessions to ensure adequate recovery.

ISOMETRIC strength training programmes

Isometric exercise involves muscle contraction against an immovable resistance. This is static exercise as tension develops in the muscle but there is no change in length. The disadvantage of isometric strength training is that strength develops only at the joint angle at which the exercise is performed and not throughout the range. This may be the requirement of some sporting activities, but if strength is required throughout the range, contractions at different points in the range must be performed.

Much research has been conducted into the effectiveness of different numbers of contractions at different percentages of maximum force. As it is difficult to judge percentages of maximum force without special apparatus, it is now accepted that it is practical to perform contractions at maximum force. It is generally agreed that substantial gains in strength will be achieved following a programme of:

5–10 maximum contractions held for 5 seconds, 3–5 days per week for 4–6 weeks.

Contractions should be performed at different points of the range, e.g.
- 5 contractions at the end of inner range
- 5 contractions at the beginning of middle range
- 5 contractions at the end of middle range
- 5 contractions at the end of outer range

Each contraction should be held for at least 5 seconds and repeated 5–10 times.

These exercises have the advantage that expensive equipment is not necessarily required. There are, however, disadvantages to isometric training.

Disadvantages of isometric resistance

■ It is difficult to ensure that the appropriate overload is applied, and to measure accurate progression.

■ Strength is developed at the point where overload is applied and therefore is not developed through the entire range.

■ There is no alternate contraction–relaxation of the muscle, therefore no pumping action to deliver blood. The maintained pressure on the capillary networks in the muscles prevents the delivery of nutrients and oxygen – fatigue will quickly develop.

■ This type of exercise raises blood pressure; isometric work should NOT be performed by anyone with heart or blood pressure problems.

ISOKINETIC strength training programmes

An isokinetic contraction develops maximum tension throughout the full range of movement. This is only possible using machines which keep the speed of movement constant.

The speed of contraction can be graded from slow to fast. Research indicates two interesting facts:

Training at slow speed will increase the strength of slow speed movements only. Training at fast speed will increase the strength of all speeds of movement. There are many routines that can be followed. One example consists of:
5 sets of 6–12 maximum contractions at fast speed 3 days/week for 6–8 weeks.

Which method is best?

Research indicates that *isokinetic* training programmes are the best for improving strength and muscle endurance. There is no muscle soreness with isokinetic work and no loss of strength. However, machines required for this work may not be available and some athletes prefer using weights which are more readily available.

Both muscle strength and endurance are also gained from *isotonic* programmes using either low repetitions and high resistance or high repetitions and low resistance. There is some degree of muscle soreness following concentric contractions but a higher level of soreness following eccentric contraction. There is also some strength loss during the recovery period.

Isometric programmes produce strength gains only at the joint angle that is exercised. Contractions should therefore be performed at three or more angles throughout the range. There is little endurance gain and there is a greater degree of muscle soreness.

Use of resistance strength training

1   To strengthen specific muscles required for sport, athletic performance, etc.

2   To improve speed and power

3   To improve muscle endurance.
4   To strengthen specific muscles for improvement of posture.
5   To generally strengthen body muscles to improve body shape.
6   To increase lean body tissue and decrease body fat.
7   To rehabilitate muscles following injury.

Planning strengthening programmes

- Assess goals, establish to what end is improvement required. The goals should be realistic and achievable, and must be discussed and agreed with the client.
- Discuss and agree a time scale.
- Assess present level of strength – this will indicate the initial starting resistance and the repetitions. Record assessment data.
- Select the training method and the equipment.
- Plan the warm-up.
- Plan the stretch routine.
- Plan the core conditioning phase.
- Plan cool-down and include some stretch.
- Consider the rest or recovery time.
- Record the load, the number of repetitions and the number of sets.

Precautions to be observed during strength training

- Set realistic objectives.
- Select weights appropriate to strength level.
- Check weights for safety.
- Start with an easy programme with light weights and few lifts.
- Perform warm-up.
- Choose a correct stable starting position.
- Secure the weights so that they cannot move or slide.
- Keep good body alignment.
- Perform the lift carefully and slowly for maximum effect with a heavy weight (momentum plays a part in fast movement – it is less effective and can result in trauma). Fast movement with low weight for endurance is safer.
- The rest between each lift should be minimal – 1–2 seconds. The rest between each set should be 1–2 minutes to allow for recovery.
- Increase number of lifts up to 30 and then increase the weight when 2–3 extra lifts can be performed.
- Do not hold the breath when lifting, as this can cause an increase in blood pressure and increases the load on the heart. Holding the breath can also increase intra-abdominal pressure which can cause hernia. Keep mouth open and breathe regularly.
- Exhale as you lift, inhale as you lower.
- Work different muscle groups. Change the exercises so that different muscles are stressed. Allow recovery time.
- Maintain a balance between agonist and antagonist.
- Replace weights and all apparatus neatly and safely.

Effects of strength training

The physiological effects of muscle strengthening are:

- The recruitment of more motor units, which increases the strength of the contraction.
- A faster neuro-muscular response, which increases the speed of contraction.
- An increase in the size and number of myofibrils, which increases strength and bulk. Recent research indicates that in some instances there may be an increase in the number of muscle fibres.
- An increase in contractile proteins myosine and actine.
- An increase in ATP, PC, enzymes and glycogen stores.
- An increase in blood flow to the muscles due to dilation (although there is no increase in the number of blood vessels or capillary networks as with endurance training).
- An increase in the mineral content of bones.
- An increase in strength of tendons and ligaments.

On average, the absolute strength in males is greater than in females. This is due to body composition and the fact that males bulk more readily than females. Research indicates that this is due to the increased presence of the male hormone testosterone, which is necessary for the synthesis of actin and myosin. However, females will develop strength in response to progressive weight training.

Muscles do not respond equally to programmes of equal intensity. The average rate of strength gain is around 5 percent per week, but some muscles gain only 1 percent, while gains of 100 percent have been recorded. Gains are greatest in the more active, fitter muscles and fast twitch fibres are more responsive to resistance training than slow twitch fibres. Improvement is greatest at the beginning of a strength training programme, levelling out as the programme continues.

Once the desired level of strength has been achieved it is easily maintained by a once weekly programme using maximum weight.

Dangers of strength training

- Muscle strain and even rupture of fibres if too much overload is applied.
- Muscle fatigue and soreness if repetitions are too high and rest periods are too short.
- Trauma – if weights are not properly secure they may fall and cause damage.
- Damage to the moving joints and their connective tissue components if the positioning of the joint is incorrect or if the lifts are casually performed.
- Overstress of other joints through poor posture and poor technique.

General strength training

These schemes include strengthening exercises for all the large muscle groups of the legs, trunk and arms. General schemes may include exercises against gravity, against one's own body weight, against resistance from a partner, or using weights such as dumb-bells, poles, ankle and wrist weights, medicine balls and so on. They may be performed individually or as a class. Exercise classes generally include some strengthening work. Circuits are also useful for general strengthening. This involves performing a number of exercises in sequence, with a set number of repetitions within a specified time.

Circuit training

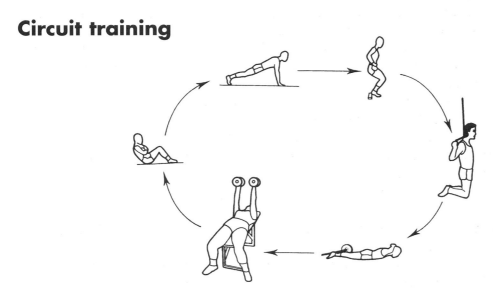

FIGURE NUMBER: 9.5 – Circuit training.

A circuit is composed of eight or more 'stations' arranged around the room. A different exercise is planned for each station. It is important to construct the circuit so that a different muscle or group of muscles is exercised at consecutive stations. This allows the muscles time to recover, preventing fatigue.

This is a very flexible form of training as the exercises can be selected to stress those systems where improvement is required.

For example, if the goal is to improve general strength then a resisted exercise for each of the large muscle groups would be selected; working one group at each station. The degree of resistance can be varied to suit the fitness level of the individual.

The programme normally consists of the initial warm up, followed by performing as many contractions as possible in 30 seconds at each station, with a break of 15–30 seconds between each station, until one circuit is complete. This is repeated until three circuits have been completed then cool down is performed.

Frequency will be three times per week for 8–10 weeks.

Decreasing the resistance but increasing the number of contractions will improve muscle endurance.

If the speed of contraction is maintained at a high level and the rest periods kept short, this programme will result in strength gains and an improvement in cardio-respiratory endurance. To improve cardio-respiratory endurance still further, some aerobic activity can be included in the programme; these are performed in between stations, e.g. skipping, walking, jogging or cycling.

If flexibility only is required then a stretch exercise would be planned at each station. If both strength and flexibility are required then both types of exercise would be included.

Circuits are very adaptable training programmes as the exercises can be selected to improve muscle strength, muscle endurance, flexibility, or cardio-respiratory endurance.

TASK

Working with a friend, role play client and therapist. Plan a circuit training programme to improve general strength for a 30-year-old female who wishes to improve body contours, before her holiday in two months time.
This could also be done as an eight week project and form part of your portfolio

---

Points to consider

- What is the goal?
- What are the time constraints?
- Which system requires improvement?
- Select the muscles that require strengthening to improve body contours.
- Organise a circuit of 8–10 exercises, one per station.
- Select exercises for different muscle groups at each station.
- Examples of strengthening exercises can be found later in this chapter.
- Use any resistance apparatus you have access to. If this is limited remember that exercises against gravity or own body weight can be included.
- Ensure that there is adequate space between station.
- Assess the client's present level of strength at each stations.
- Use a resistance of 60–66 percent 1 RM.
- Teach each exercise, making sure that the client understands what is required and is performing it correctly before starting the programme.
- Explain that she is to perform as many contractions as possible in 30 seconds but they must be accurately performed. Accuracy must not be sacrificed for speed. She should rest for 30 seconds between each station or longer if there are signs of stress such as breathlessness, profuse sweating or extreme reddening. She may complete the circuit 2 or 3 times depending on her stress level. Keep accurate records of weights used, client weight and muscle girth measurement. Check progress each week that there were no adverse effects. Stress the importance of attending regularly, for example, 3 times per week.

QUESTIONS

1. Explain briefly what is meant by cardio-respiratory fitness.
2. At what level of intensity should an individual exercise in order to improve cardio-respiratory endurance?
3. Explain briefly how you would calculate an individual's maximum heart rate.
4. At what percentage of maximum heart rate should a beginner exercise?
5. List ten important effects of endurance training.
6. Define the following terms
   a Muscle strength
   b Muscle endurance
7. Explain what is meant by the term 'One repetition maximum'.
8. List four disadvantages of isometric strength training.
9. Explain briefly how you would construct a circuit for strengthening the large muscle groups of the legs and arms. Name the muscles and explain the selected exercise.
10. List six effects of muscle strength training.
11. Explain the principal difference between training for muscle strength and muscle endurance.
12. Explain the following principles of training: specificity, overload, progression, training threshold.

LEARN

The maximum weight that can be lifted by a muscle just once is known as one repetition maximum (1 RM).

LEARN

For strength training, a muscle must be made to lift over 66 percent of 1 RM

It is essential to keep accurate records of the programme and progress.

The following data must be recorded on a record card.

Weight selected over 66% of 1 RM up to 85–95% of 1 RM	No of repetitions 6–10	No. of sets 3–5 with full recovery in between

TASK

Work with a partner. One person should sit in a high sitting position, with thighs supported and feet off the floor. Assess 3 RM for the quadriceps muscle. (This is the maximum weight that can be lifted 3 times.) Strap increasing weights around the ankles until the appropriate weight is reached. The foot should be dorsi-flexed, and the knee must straighten maximally and lock at the end of each lift.

The pyramid method

This is effective for strength, bulk and endurance. As the weight increases the repetitions decrease. For example, a client might perform five repetitions at 2 kg, four at 3 kg, three at 4 kg and two at 5 kg, and then reverse the order, reducing the weight and increasing the repetitions. The maximum weight that can be lifted twice is assessed, and the pyramid is constructed from that starting point. A one-sided regime is sometimes used, working up to maximum weight and then resting.

LEARN

Muscle endurance is the ability of a muscle to contract continuously over a period of time

Muscle endurance

This is the ability of the muscles to perform repeated contractions continuously over a period of time. The main difference in training for endurance as opposed to training for strength is that lighter weights are used and the repetitions are increased. The method employed is the same.

Endurance training

Weight selected	No. of Repetitions	Sets
under 60% of 1 RM	20–30–50	3
from 40–60% 1 RM		

For endurance, the weight is kept below 66 per cent of the maximum and repeated 25–50 times or more. Training must be repeated 3–5 times per week.

- Speed can be improved using high-speed contractions with low resistance.
- To increase power (speed × strength), 3 sets of 15 high-speed contractions with 30–60 per cent of maximal load is generally recommended.

The effects of muscle endurance training

The physiological effects of training for endurance are:

- an increase in the number and size of blood vessels in the muscles;
- an increase in the number of capillary networks;
- an increase in the number of mitochondria in the muscle cells;
- an increase in the number of oxidative enzymes, which extract oxygen from the blood – the aerobic capacity of the muscles is therefore improved;
- an increase in glycogen stores and glycolitic enzymes used for energy.

Plyometrics

Explosive power will improve using *plyometrics*. These are jumping, leaping and hopping movements, where the prime mover is stretched before contraction. The speed of the stretch is an important factor. When a muscle is stretched, the stretch receptors within the muscle are stimulated. This increases the strength of the following contraction. The longer and faster the stretch, the greater the following concentric contraction. There is a danger of damaging joints and producing micro-tears in muscle fibres when performing these exercises. They must only be performed by the very fit and only after adequate warm-up.

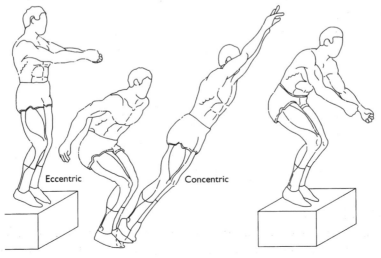

Eccentric   Concentric

FIGURE NUMBER: 9.6 – Plyometric training.

> **LEARN**
> For endurance training the weight is kept below 66 percent of 1RM but repetitions are high, 20–50 lifts

Summary and aid to learning

Fitness means having the energy and skill to cope in one's environment.

This obviously means different things to different people. For some people it simply means coping with the tasks of daily living but at the other end of the scale, for the athlete, it will mean performing skills at the highest level.

When we consider training for improving fitness we must ask two questions:
- Fitness for what? (what is the desired outcome?)
- Where are we starting from? (what is the present level of fitness?)

We can improve fitness by considering all the factors that contribute to fitness.

Cardio-respiratory endurance means improving the condition of the heart and lungs, thus improving the delivery of nutrients and oxygen to the tissue cells.

Muscle strength means the maximal force a muscle can develop against resistance which will make activities easier.

Muscle endurance means improving the ability of muscles to contract for longer periods.

Flexibility means improving the suppleness of connective tissue components within the muscles which will improve extensibility and elasticity. It also improves the tensile strength and extensibility of ligaments and tendons. These factors will enable the tissues to withstand excessive forces, reducing the likelihood of injury.

Skill refers to accurate performance with little or no waste of energy. It is largely a function of the nervous system which initiates, controls and coordinates all activities.

Speed refers to the distance moved in a specific time. Some activities will require fast speed while others require slow control. Speed is an important factor in most sport because improved speed and strength will result in greater power.

Body composition refers to the ratio of body fat and fat-free tissue. It is dependent on energy balance which is the balance between energy consumed (the food eaten), and energy expended (the amount of activity undertaken).

Nutrition refers to the foods we eat and the role they play in sustaining life. Good nutrition means eating the required amount of a variety of foods which will enable the body to function at maximum efficiency.

Rest and relaxation means allowing the body sufficient time to recover following activity. The more intense the activity the longer the rest period should be. Many physiological improvements continue into the rest period. Adequate rest will prevent chronic fatigue.

Relaxation means freedom from stress and is related to rest. Stress adversly affects the function of many body systems. Consequently reducing stress factors will enable the body to function more efficiently.

Planning programmes

The following **principles of training** must be considered when planning a training programme:

Specificity means that the programme must be specific to the component or systems that require improving, e.g. muscle strength.

Overload means that the training load must be greater than that normally encountered.

Progression means that the overload must be progressively increased in line with improvement. The work must become harder as improvement is gained.

Training threshold is the minimum intensity of exercise required to gain improvement.

Reversibility refers to the fact that training gains will regress when training stops.

Cardio-respiratory endurance

Also known as **aerobic capacity or endurance**, this refers to the capability of the lungs to take in adequate oxygen and the ability of the heart to deliver it to the muscles.

Any form of low intensity, long duration activity, performed over a period of time will improve endurance.

Select four activities which will improve aerobic endurance.

Intensity

The intensity must be greater than that normally encountered. The heart rate/pulse rate is used to establish the appropriate intensity.

An individual must not exercise above their maximum heart rate. To determine **maximum heart rate** deduct the person's age from 220.

The maximum heart rate for a 30 year old would be 190 beats per minute. The heart rate must not rise above this during training. However, to produce a training effect the person must exercise at above 60 per cent of this maximum heart rate but this can increase to 90 per cent as fitness develops; this is the **target zone**. The rate which should be maintained throughout the session is known as *the target rate*.

Calculate the target rate for a 30 year old exercising at 60 per cent of maximum heart rate.

Frequency

This refers to the number of training sessions per week; for endurance this will be 4–5 times per week.

Duration

This can refer to two things:

- the duration of each session for endurance must be over 30 minutes; it is usually longer.
- the duration of the training programme – for endurance this will be 12–16 weeks.

Following an endurance training programme one would expect an improvement in the physiological functioning of the lungs, the heart and blood, and of the muscles. Study the text and write a list of these improvements.

Endurance training improves the capacity to use fat as fuel, therefore a programme of endurance training and a controlled diet is the best way of reducing body fat.

Muscle strength

This refers to the maximal force a muscle can develop against resistance. Strength is measured by the maximum weight a muscle can lift. This is known as one repetition maximum (1 RM).

Strength improves in response to lifting increasing loads; this is refered to as weight training.

The principles of weight training programmes are:

Overload means that the overload must be more than is generally encountered. It must be over 66 per cent of 1 RM.

Progression means the load must be increased as strength develops.

Arrangement of the exercises means successive exercises should not work the same muscle.

Specificity means the exercises must target the specific muscles where strength is required.

Recovery means the muscles must be given time to recover, both between sets and between training days. Overtraining without adequate rest can result in chronic fatigue.

Although weight training usually refers to isotonic contraction, both isometric and isokinetic contractions can be used.

Explain the difference between these types of contraction.

Strength gains are achieved using a low number of contractions but high resistance. Bulk will increase with strength but one or two lifts at maximum load should be included.

A programme might include 6–10 contractions grouped into a set; if 1–5 sets are performed the duration will be 6–10 weeks. This is just one example. The numbers can be varied slightly to suit the individual and type of contraction.

Muscle endurance refers to the ability of a muscle to continue contracting over a long period of time.

To improve muscle endurance the programme will involve high repetitions and low resistance.

A programme might include 30–50 repetitions of low weight between 40–60 per cent of 1 RM, frequency 3 times per week for 6–10 weeks.

Muscle power is a product of strength and speed and is a requirement of some sports. This is achieved through plyometric training which includes jumping, leaping and hopping movements where the prime mover is stretched before contraction.

STRENGTHENING EXERCISES

Calf strengthening exercises

NAME: GASTROCNEMIUS, SOLEUS ACTION: PLANTAR FLEXORS
POSITION: CALF MUSCLES

Starting position	Exercise
■ Standing	lift up onto toes and down.
■ Standing on one leg	lift up onto toes and down. Repeat with other leg.
■ Standing	step onto a step, then lift onto toes. Repeat with other leg.

When these three exercises become too easy and the client can perform 20–30 without difficulty, weights can be used to increase the effort. Hold equal weights in each hand, beginning with 1 kg and increasing gradually as muscle strength improves.

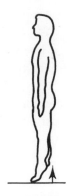

FIGURE NUMBER: 9.7

■ Long sitting with resistance rubber belt around the feet held by hand

push both feet against the belt, then push alternate feet against the belt.
or
use multigym and plantar flex against the resistance.

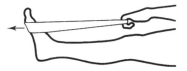

FIGURE NUMBER: 9.8

The following activities will also improve the strength and mobility of the foot and ankle:
■ Walking: push off onto toes
■ Jumping: pushing from toes
■ Hop on one foot and then the other
■ Skip on the toes
■ Sprint from one wall to another
■ Run or jog on a flat surface
■ Run or jog up a hill
■ Jump across a bench, either with bunny jumps or straight.

Quadriceps strengthening exercises

NAME: RECTUS FEMORIS, VASTUS MEDIALIS, VASTUS LATERALIS, VASTUS INTERMEDIUS
ACTION: KNEE EXTENSORS
POSITION: FRONT OF THIGH

Starting position	Exercise
■ Long sitting	press the back of the knee down into the bed and tighten the quadriceps muscle: dorsi-flex the foot and try to lift the heel just off the bed. Hold and release.
■ Long sitting with a rolled towel under the heel	press the back of the knee downwards and tighten the quadriceps muscle; dorsi-flex the foot. Hold and release.
■ Long sitting	dorsi-flex the foot and tighten the knee. Raise the leg just off the bed keeping the knee tight and straight.

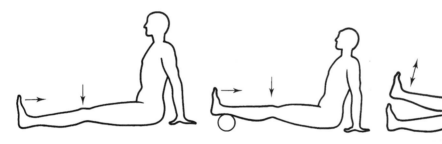

FIGURE NUMBER: 9.9   **FIGURE NUMBER: 9.10**   **FIGURE NUMBER: 9.11**

If the knee bends slightly it indicates that the muscle is weak and that the above exercises must be continued until the leg can be lifted without any give.

■ Long sitting	dorsi-flex the foot and tighten the knee, then lift the leg and circle it slowly around.
■ Long sitting	dorsi-flex the foot and tighten the knee, lift the leg and lower it almost to the bed, then lift it again several times.

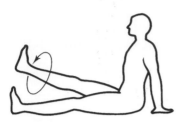

FIGURE NUMBER: 9.12

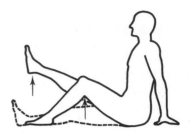

FIGURE NUMBER: 9.13

■ Long sitting

dorsi-flex the foot and tighten the knee, lift the leg and swing it out sideways. Repeat several times.

■ Long sitting with tightly rolled towel behind knee under thigh

dorsi-flex the foot and lift the lower leg to straighten the knee, then lower.

■ Crook sitting

straighten alternate legs, keeping thighs parallel.

■ Long sitting with a weight across the ankle

dorsi-flex the foot, keeping the heel clear of the ground as the knee is tightened. Then lift the leg and weight off the bed. Hold and lower. (Do not lift too high – 24 cm is enough.) Begin with a weight that can just be lifted with a straight knee.

■ Long sitting with rolled towel behind the knee, weight over ankle as above

press the back of the knee into the towel and straighten the knee, Hold and release.

■ High sitting on a high chair or on the edge of a couch, feet off the floor and knee at 90°. Weight strapped to ankle as above.

Slowly lift the weight until the knee is straight. Keep the thigh in contact with the couch. Hold and lower slowly back to 90° bend. Repeat ten times, then rest for one minute. Repeat again until weight is lifted 30 times. Then increase weight. If the knee cannot fully straighten, the weight is too great. Repeat with a lower weight.

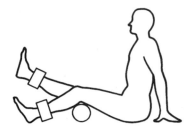

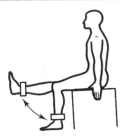

FIGURE NUMBER: 9.14   **FIGURE NUMBER: 9.15**

This last exercise can be performed with an elasticated band or spring attached to the chair, level with the ankle, against which the leg then pulls. Use a leg-press machine if available.

Note: before using weights to improve strength, read the notes on weight training earlier in this chapter.

■ Wing standing	bend the knees and lower the body slowly, bending to just above a right angle. Keep the back straight. Push up straight and lock the knees by pulling patella upwards. (Caution: do not take the buttocks below knee level.)

This can be progressed by holding a weight in the arms or by placing them over the shoulders. A fit person could perform this with one leg at a time.

■ Using a multigym or sliding sprung board or rowing machine	bend the knees fully. Then push out to straighten and tighten the knees, hold it and bend the knees again slowly. Keep the back straight.
■ Standing in front of a bench or stairs	step up, straighten the knee fully, then step down. Do ten or more per leg. A fit person could step up and down two stairs at a time.

Cycling is also beneficial to the quadriceps muscle. Make sure that the leg can straighten during each downward movement of the pedal. To progress, increase the resistance as necessary on an exercise bike or cycle uphill on an ordinary bicycle.

Hamstring strengthening exercises

NAME: BICEPS FEMORIS, SEMIMEMBRANOSUS, SEMITENDINOSUS
ACTION: KNEE FLEXORS AND HIP EXTENSORS
POSITION: BACK OF THIGH

Starting position	*Exercise*
■ High sitting with heel resting on floor	press alternate heels into the floor.
■ High sitting with heels against the chair legs	press the back of the heel alternately into the chair legs. Progress by sitting forward so that the knee is bent to a greater angle.
■ Standing	bend alternate knees to a right angle and extend the hip (push it backwards).
■ Standing with weight around ankles	bend alternate knees to a right angle and extend the hip. Progress by extending with a straight leg.
■ Prone lying	cross the legs at the ankles, bend the leg underneath and resist with leg on top.
■ Prone lying with weights around ankle	bend alternate knees to a right angle and lift the leg upwards from the hip.
■ Prone lying with bent knees, with an elastic strap or spring tied to the ankle and behind at ankle level, or use a multigym	bend the knee to a right angle against the resistance.

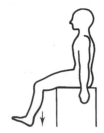

FIGURE NUMBER: 9.16

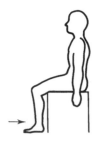

FIGURE NUMBER: 9.17

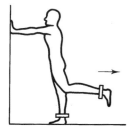

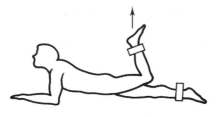

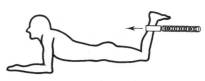

FIGURE NUMBER: 9.18   **FIGURE NUMBER: 9.19**   **FIGURE NUMBER: 9.20**

Hip extensor strengthening exercises

NAME: GLUTEUS MAXIMUS ACTION: HIP EXTENSOR
POSITION: BUTTOCK

Starting position	Exercise
■ Supine lying or high sitting	tighten buttocks, then release.
■ Supine lying	tighten buttocks and lift slightly off the floor.
■ Crook lying	lift buttocks off the floor. do not hyper extend the back.
■ Standing	swing alternate legs forwards and backwards, lowering slowly.
■ Stride standing	slide arms down the legs, bend trunk forwards and return to upright.
■ Standing with weights on ankles	swing alternate legs backwards and lower slowly.
■ Standing with weights on ankles	bend the knee to a right angle and press the leg backwards with short movements.
■ High sitting	stand up and sit down slowly.
■ High sitting	press the thighs downwards into the seat and rotate them outwards.
■ Prone lying	bend alternate knees and lift the leg off the floor. (Caution: keep the hips against the floor.) Ankle weights can be used for progression.

- Prone lying

  lift alternate legs off the floor. (Caution: keep the hips against the floor.)

- Prone kneeling

  lift leg backwards and upwards (ankle weights can be used for progression).

- Prone lying with weights around ankle

  lift alternate legs off the floor.

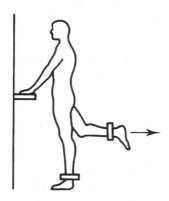

FIGURE NUMBER: 9.21

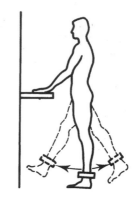

FIGURE NUMBER: 9.22

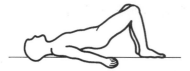

FIGURE NUMBER: 9.23

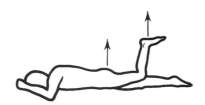

FIGURE NUMBER: 9.24

- Stoop standing with trunk supported on the bed

  raise alternate legs backwards and upwards. Keep the knee straight and the hips on the bed. Ankle weights can be used for progression.

- Prone lying on couch with one leg over the edge

  lift the hanging leg backwards and upwards. Repeat with the other leg. Repeat with weights around the ankles.

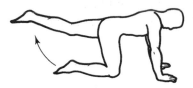

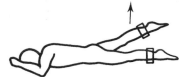

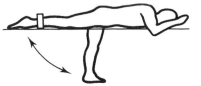

FIGURE NUMBER: 9.25   **FIGURE NUMBER: 9.26**   **FIGURE NUMBER: 9.27**

Abductor strengthening exercises

NAME: GLUTUS MEDIUS, GLUTEUS MINIMUS AND TENSOR FASCIA LATA
ACTION: HIP ABDUCTORS AND MEDIAL ROTATORS
POSITION: LATERAL ASPECT OF HIP AND THIGH

Starting position	*Exercise*
■ Supine lying	part the legs and then close them.
■ Supine lying	lift alternate legs slightly, move them out to the side and return to the centre.
■ High sitting or lying with feet inside the legs of a chair	push both legs outwards against the legs of the chair, hold, then release.
■ As above	use a partner and push against his or her legs.
■ Support standing	keeping the back straight, swing alternate legs slowly out sideways and back. Occasionally hold the leg in abduction.
■ Support standing with weights on ankles	as above, swing alternate legs slowly out sideways and back. Hold in abduction.
■ Side lying with underneath leg bent for balance	lift the upper leg, hold and lower. Keep the hip pushed forwards throughout. Progress using weights.

Note: when this last exercise is performed correctly only 35–40° of abduction is possible, due to the structure of the joint. Individuals may gain greater range by rolling the hip backwards, but this brings the hip flexors into play and therefore does not work the abductors.

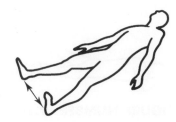

FIGURE NUMBER: 9.28

■ Side lying with weight on elbow	push the pelvis upwards to arch away from the floor.

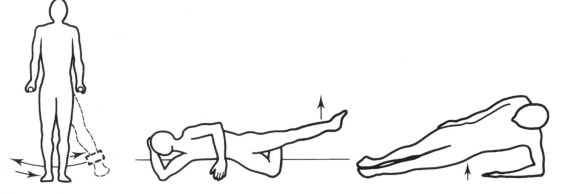

FIGURE NUMBER: 9.29   **FIGURE NUMBER: 9.30**   **FIGURE NUMBER: 9.31**

Adductor strengthening exercises

NAME: ADDUCTOR MAGNUS, ADDUCTOR LONGUS, ADDUCTOR BREVIS, PECTINEUS AND GRACILIS: ACTION: HIP ADDUCTORS AND LATERAL ROTATORS
POSITION: MEDIAL ASPECT OF THIGH

Starting position	Exercise
■ Supine lying	part the legs and then close them.
■ Supine lying	lift alternate legs slightly, move them out to the side and then back across the other leg.
■ Supine lying	bend the knees onto the chest and then straighten the legs into the air, keeping them at 90°. Scissor the legs open and across.
■ High sitting or lying with feet outside the legs of a chair	push both legs inwards against the legs of the chair, hold and release.

■ As above	use a partner and push against his or her legs.
■ Crook lying	part the knees and then close them. Repeat with the hands on the inside of the knees, pushing against the movement.
■ Crook lying	place a pillow or firm sponge between the knees and press the knees together.
■ Support standing	keeping the back straight, swing alternate legs out slowly sideways and return across the other leg, hold and release.
■ Support standing with weights on ankles	as above, swing alternate legs out slowly sideways and return slowly across the other leg, hold and release.
■ Side lying with upper leg bent	raise lower leg upwards, hold and release. Progress by using heavier weights.

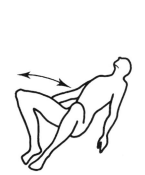
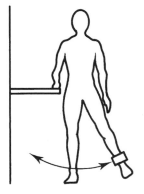
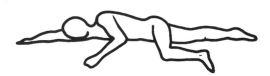

FIGURE NUMBER: 9.32   **FIGURE NUMBER: 9.33**   **FIGURE NUMBER: 9.34**

Abdominal strengthening exercises

NAME: RECTUS ABDOMINUS, EXTERNAL OBLIQUE, INTERNAL OBLIQUE, TRANSVERSUS ABDOMINUS
ACTION: TRUNK FLEXORS, SIDE FLEXORS AND ROTATORS
POSITION: COVER THE ABDOMEN

Starting position	Exercise
■ Crook lying	press the small of the back into the floor, tilt the pelvis backwards and pull the stomach in. Hold and release.
■ Crook lying	press the small of the back into the floor. Tuck the head down onto the chest, then raise the head and shoulders to look at the knees. Hold and release.
■ Crook lying	bring both knees up to form right angles at hip and knee. Reach up towards the ceiling with alternate knees.
■ Crook lying, arms at side	curl up (Caution: return slowly from the base of the spine upwards.)
■ Crook lying, arms across chest	curl up.
■ Crook lying, hands on shoulders	curl up.
■ Crook lying, hands on ears	curl up. (Do not put the hands behind the neck as this can damage the neck.)
■ Stretch crook lying	curl up. (Caution: only for those with strong abdominals.) Keep the arms back: do not swing them forwards.
■ Crook lying, holding a weight or medicine ball on the chest	curl up. (Caution: only for those with strong abdominals.)

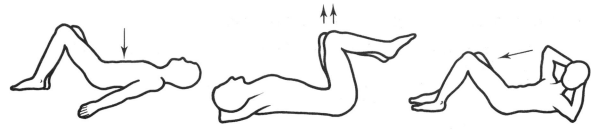

FIGURE NUMBER: 9.35   **FIGURE NUMBER: 9.36**   **FIGURE NUMBER: 9.37**

■ Crook lying, hands on shoulders	twist to turn the right elbow towards the left knee, return and repeat with the opposite side.
■ Crook lying	keep knees together drop to right & left.
■ Crook lying	bend the knees onto the chest and then stretch the legs towards the ceiling. Reach upwards to the ceiling with the feet.
■ Crook lying	bend the knees onto the chest and then stretch the legs towards the ceiling. Keeping the feet together make small circles in the air.

Back strengthening exercises

NAME: ERECTOR SPINAE, QUADRATUS LUMBORUM
ACTION: BACK EXTENSORS AND SIDE FLEXORS
POSITION: COVER THE BACK

Starting position	*Exercise*
■ Prone lying	lift alternate legs and lower.
■ Stretch prone lying	lift alternate arms and lower.
■ Stretch prone lying	stretch the left arm and right leg along the floor, then lift them slightly and release. Repeat with the other arm and leg.
■ Prone lying, arms to sides	keeping the chin in to the chest, lift the head and shoulders, then lower slowly.

■ Prone lying, hands clasped behind back	keeping the chin in and the elbows straight, lift the head and shoulders, then lower them slowly.
■ Stretch prone lying	keeping the chin in, lift the arms, head and shoulders, then lower them slowly. This may be progressed by holding weights in the hands.
■ Prone lying, arms to side, with the head and shoulders over the edge of the bed (fix the feet)	lift the head and shoulders as high as possible, then slowly lower them.
■ As above with hands on shoulders	lift the arms, head and shoulders as high as possible, then slowly lower them.

Note: these exercises should not be undertaken by anyone with back problems or pain.

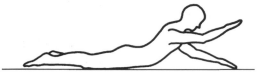

FIGURE NUMBER: 9.38

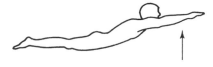

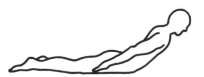

FIGURE NUMBER: 9.39　　　　**FIGURE NUMBER: 9.40**

Trapezius and rhomboid strengthening exercises

ACTION: RETRACTORS OF THE SHOULDER GIRDLE
POSITION: COVER UPPER BACK

Starting position	Exercise
■ Stride standing	circle the shoulders backwards alternately and then together.
■ Stride standing	pull the shoulders down and backwards.
■ Across bend stride standing	pull the elbows backwards and release, then straighten the arms and pull backwards.

This last exercise, commonly called 'pull pull fling', should be done slowly and deliberately, as too fast a movement activates the stretch reflex within the antagonistic muscle and may result in micro-tears of the myofibrils (see chapter 7).

■ Standing with heels 10 cm away from wall	flatten the back against the wall and stretch the arms above the head, palms facing forward. Keeping the back against the wall, slide the arms down along the wall, bending the elbows. Slide the arms up and down the wall.
■ High sitting, hands on thighs	bend forward with the chest to the thighs. Raise the trunk inch by inch, pushing shoulders into the back of the chair.
■ High sitting	bend forward as above, but raise the trunk against the resistance of a therapist applying force behind the shoulders.
■ Prone lying	keeping the chin in, raise the head and shoulders off the floor, hold and release, then lower slowly.
■ Prone lying, hands clasped behind back	keeping the chin in, pull the shoulders back and lift the head and shoulders off the floor. Hold and lower slowly.
■ Prone lying, hands on shoulders	keeping the chin in, pull the shoulders back and lift the head and shoulders off the floor. Hold and lower slowly.
■ Yard prone lying	keeping the chin in, lift the arms backwards and raise the head and shoulders off the floor.

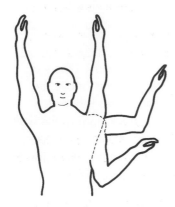

FIGURE NUMBER: 9.42

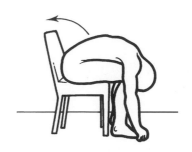

FIGURE NUMBER: 9.43

Serratus anterior and Triceps strengthening exercises

NAME: SERRATUS ANTERIOR
POSITION: UNDER SCAPULA
NAME: TRICEPS
POSITION: POSTERIOR ASPECT OF UPPER ARM
ACTION: POSITIONING OF SCAPULA DURING MOVEMENTS OF THE ARM AND
HOLDING THE SCAPULA AGAINST THE CHEST WALL. THE SAME EXERCISES ARE USED
FOR THE EXTENSOR OF THE ELBOW TRICEPS

Starting position	*Exercise*
■ Across bend stride standing	pull the elbows back and straighten the arms out to the side slowly and delibrately.
■ Bend stride standing	punch the air, a pillow, a punch bag or the therapist's hands.
■ Bend stride standing	push forwards against the resistance of the therapist, first with both hands, then alternately.
■ Bend stride standing	straighten the arms up above the head alternately and then together.
■ Stride standing or high sitting	lean the body forwards, straighten the arms and stretch them backwards. (Hand weights can be used for progression.)
■ Stride standing, arms bent, hands on wall	push the body away from the wall by straightening the elbows.

■ Prone kneeling	bend and straighten the elbows.
■ Prone lying	bend and straighten the elbows, lifting the upper trunk (half press-up).
■ Prone lying	press-up.
■ Crook lying, holding weights in hands at shoulder level	push the weights vertically upwards and lower them, first alternately, then together. Progress by increasing the weights.
■ Yard crook lying	holding the weights, raise the arms from the side to ceiling. Progress by increasing the weights.

These exercises should not be performed by a client with round shoulders as they strengthen the pectoral muscles.

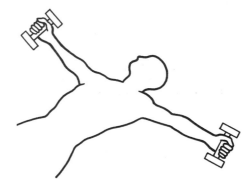

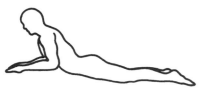

FIGURE NUMBER: 9.44

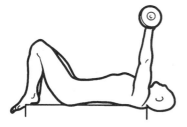

FIGURE NUMBER: 9.45

FIGURE NUMBER: 9.46

TASKS

Select exercises from the previous list, and add any of your own:
■ Devise exercise schemes for strengthening the following muscles – gastrocnemius; quadriceps; hamstrings; gluteus maximus; abductors; adductors; abdominals; the middle fibres of the trapezius; rhomboids.
■ Teach one of your schemes to a partner or group.

IMPROVING FLEXIBILITY OR SUPPLENESS

This refers to the range of movement possible at a joint or group of joints. A joint will move through an arc of movement from one point to another, for example from full flexion to full extension. (See chapter 3.)

> **LEARN**
> Flexibility refers to the range of movement possible at a joint or group of joints

Joints must be considered separately, as flexibility is specific to each joint. However, an activity such as throwing a ball will require flexibility at more than one joint, and therefore the movement at all of those joints must be considered. Flexibility can be increased through regular training and will contribute to efficient technique, improved performance and the prevention of injury. There are a number of factors that influence or limit flexibility:

- Joint structure
- Age
- Sex
- Body temperature
- Strength training.

Joint structure

This is the main factor influencing flexibility. It includes:

- the shape and contour of the articulating surfaces (the tighter the fit the more limited the range).
- the tension of the connective tissue components, the capsule and supporting ligaments; and the connective tissue within and around the muscles.
- the tension of the muscles and tendons acting on and surrounding the joint. Flexibility will be limited by voluntary or reflex contraction of the muscles acting joint. When a muscle is stretched to its limit, the muscle spindles located in the muscle are activated. These sensory receptors transmit impulses to the spinal cord and a reflex contraction of the muscle occurs. This is a protective mechanism to prevent further stretch which could damage the muscle. Pulling against this contraction may result in tears of the muscle.

Age

Generally, ageing reduces flexibility, but training and activity will influence the degree of loss. Young children are very flexible and, depending on the level of activity, this flexibility continues to increase up to adolescence at around 15 years of age. After the age of 15 there is a natural decrease in flexibility. The rate of decrease will depend upon the training, exercise and activities practised by the individual. Research indicates that flexibility can be increased for all age groups if appropriate exercises are undertaken, but the rate of increase will be greater in younger age groups and will decline with age.

Training

As stated above, training and the selection of appropriate exercise will increase flexibility for all age groups. Those individuals, such as gymnasts and ballet dancers, who continue with uninterrupted training programmes will have greater flexibility than the untrained.

Sex (Gender)

It has been suggested that females are more flexible than males, although the evidence is inconclusive. Females on the whole have lighter and smaller bones, which may influence flexibility. In the main they have a shorter leg length and lower centre of gravity, making certain movements easier. They are also designed for flexibility of the pelvic region to facilitate childbirth.

Body temperature

The elevation of body temperature increases flexibility. Therefore, warm-up exercises must be performed before flexibility training. Pre-heating with hot packs, heat lamps, hot baths or showers, diathermy or massage will increase the effect. These methods may be used before warm-up but not instead of exercises. The heat reduces viscosity and relaxes tissues, which thus offer less resistance to movement. Heat also increases the extensibility of connective and muscle tissue surrounding the joint.

Strength training

Certain strength training routines can limit joint flexibility. Strength training must be planned to include full-range movements and eccentric work.

In the same way as we overload a muscle in order to increase strength, we must overstretch in order to increase flexibility. The body continually adapts to increasing demand placed upon it, so that moving a joint beyond its existing range and stretching the surrounding tissues will result in increased range as the tissues become more extensible.

Uses of stretching exercises

Stretching increases the range of movement and will improve the performance of simple activities required for daily living and also the complex activities required by the elite performer.

Stretching increases the suppleness and range of the tissues and joints, enabling them to accommodate any increased stresses; this will reduce the risk of injury.

Gentle, uniform stretching eases tension and spasm which reduces pain and stiffness.

Stretching of tight muscles will improve muscle balance which will contribute to good posture.

Stretching is an important part of the rehabilitation following injury. The healing process may result in the formation of scar tissue within the muscle. This must be kept supple and its elasticity maintained, otherwise it will contract and impair the contractile properties of the muscle.

Stretching exercises should aways be included in any exercise scheme. They should be practised after the warm-up in order to enhance performance and reduce the risk of injury. They should be performed during the cool-down to reduce muscle soreness and stiffness. Stretching exercises can also be used as a complete programme, designed progressively to increase the range in all body joints. This type of slow stretch programme allows time for thought and meditation and, as in yoga, pursues a harmony of body, mind and spirit.

Methods of stretching

There are various methods of stretching, including ballistic, dynamic, static, proprioceptive neuro-muscular facilitation (PNF) and others.

Ballistic stretching

This type of stretching involves fast, jerky movements where the increased momentum created by a 'bounce' is used to increase movement at the end of the range, for example bouncing to touch the toes. Ballistics are not generally recommended and should be avoided in class work.

The arguments against their use are physiologically sound:
- A quick or rapid stretch does not allow sufficient time for the tissues to adapt, resulting in strain.
- A sudden jerk applied to a muscle will initiate the stretch reflex and muscle tension will increase. Further pulling against this tension may result in microscopic tears of the myofibrils. Healing will result in the formation of fibrous scar tissue, which impairs the function of the muscle.
- A quick stretch does not allow for neurological adaptation. Research has shown that the tension generated in a muscle by a fast stretch is far greater than that generated by a slow stretch. Therefore the tensile resistance to fast stretching is much greater.
- Bouncing movements are not easy to control. Therefore the positioning of joints and the direction of movement may not be correct, increasing the likelihood of injury.

> **LEARN**
> Ballistic stretching is not recommended and should be avoided. Jerking may result in tears of myofibrils which will impair muscle function.

Despite all these reasons for not attempting ballistics, some people favour their use for specific training. There is some evidence that following ballistic or fast stretch training the stretch reflex may be delayed and will be activated nearer the end of range of movement, thus improving performance. Gymnasts and dancers may include ballistic exercises prior to specific actions or routines, but generally they should be avoided.

Dynamic stretching

These are movements where a muscle or muscles are worked gradually through their range. Beginning with short-range movements, the actions move progressively through to maximum full range. Dynamic flexibility is required by ball kickers in rugby and soccer, e.g. a gradual stretching of the hamstrings in stages before kicking ensures that the effort of the muscles kicking the ball is not hampered by tight hamstrings. Repetitive free knee extension is performed, increasing the range each time.

Static stretching

These are movements which take a muscle slowly and deliberately to the end of its range. The position is then held and further stretch applied. During the holding time, the muscle adapts to the stretch. The stretch reflex controlled by the muscle spindles is inhibited, there is a slow decrease in muscle tension and the muscle relaxes. This allows an increase in muscle length and in the range of joint movement. Research has shown that low-force, long-duration stretching at a raised temperature will result in permanent lengthening.

Static stretching is safer and more effective than ballistic or dynamic stretching, as the tissues have time to relax. Maximum stretch is achieved when a muscle is fully relaxed and connective tissue is fully stretched. The stretch reflex is inhibited, and so there is no risk of tearing, muscle soreness and damage. Movements are slower, more controlled and more functionally accurate, and there is therefore less risk of injury. Static stretching requires less energy consumption.

Static stretching may be classified into active and passive stretching.
- Active stretching is stretching alone, without external aid.
- Active assisted stretching is a stretch performed alone until a limit is reached, at which point a partner helps to gain a further stretch.
- Passive stretching is achieved by an external force such as traction or a partner, while the individual remains inactive.

All static stretching must be controlled and performed with care. Particular care, effective communication and trust must exist between partners in active assisted and passive stretching. These should only be practised by competent, well-trained individuals.

Proprioceptive neuromuscular facilitation

There are many PNF techniques, which are an excellent way of increasing range of movement, but they require an in-depth knowledge of neurophysiology and are not within the scope of this book. However, one of the techniques, *alternate contract/relax*, is straightforward and useful, especially following recovery from injury.

This form of increased range is achieved in the following way.

A muscle is moved to its point of slight stretch, i.e. at the end of joint movement, and an isometric contraction of that muscle against resistance is performed and held. This is followed by relaxation and further joint movement, which will now be possible.

For example, in prone lying (face down), lift one leg to stretch the hip flexors. Ask a partner to support the leg and to resist an isometric contraction (i.e. not to allow movement as you push down against his or her hand). Relax, then lift the leg higher, as the hip flexors will now allow a greater range of movement.

In sitting, tilt the head to the left to stretch the right sterno-cleido-mastoid. Now place the hand against the right side of the face. Contract the muscle statically against the hand resistance, hold and relax. The head will now move further to the left.

Techniques of static stretching

- Select a suitable venue that is warm and well ventilated. Ensure that there is sufficient space to perform all movements.
- Wear warm clothing to maintain and increase body temperature.
- Check that the floor surface is clean, smooth and non-slip.
- Do not stretch if any of the following contra-indications are present: hyper-mobility, strains or sprains, inflammation of joints, pain in joints, fevers, heart problems, high or low blood pressure, or after a heavy meal.
- Identify the goals (where flexibility is required). Always warm up with a set of exercises designed to work the large muscle groups. This warm-up will increase muscle temperature, reduce muscle viscosity, decrease muscle tension and promote relaxation and will make tissues more extensible.
- Set the mind into a tranquil and relaxed state.
- Isolate the muscle or group for stretching and place the joint in the correct position. Stretch slowly and evenly, feeling the pull in the belly of the muscle and not at the tendon ends. There should be a feeling of mild discomfort, not pain. Hold the stretch for six to ten seconds to begin with, increasing to 20–30 seconds over time. As the tension decreases, stretch a little further – do not jerk or bounce at the end of the movement. Let pain be the guide. If the pain increases, relax; if the muscle begins to quiver, relax; if muscle tension increases, relax. Move slowly out of the stretch.
- Repeat the stretch five times at the beginning of a programme, eventually working up to ten to fifteen repetitions.
- Exhale as you move into the stretch and relax.
- Stretching programmes should be performed once or twice a day if rapid improvement is required.

The effects of stretch training

The physiological effects of flexibility training are:

- an increased range of movement at joints;

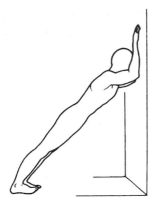

FIGURE NUMBER: 9.47 –
Active stretch for the gastrocenius.

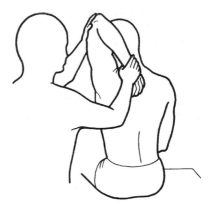

FIGURE NUMBER: 9.48 –
Active assisted stretching of triceps.

- increased flexibility of the supporting structures;
- increased elasticity and extensibility of muscles;
- reduced tension and increased relaxation in the muscles;
- increased circulation to the muscles;
- improved balance and co-ordination between muscle groups;
- improved posture;
- improved mechanical efficiency and improved speed and skill;
- improved techique and performance, since relaxation of the antagonistic muscles allows the agonist to maximise performance;
- neurological adaptation delaying the stretch reflex;
- if performed after performance, particularly eccentric work, a reduction of muscle soreness.

Dangers of stretching exercises

- Damage to muscles by causing micro-tears of muscle fibres, caused by sudden stretch of cold muscles, or ballistrics;
- Damage to joints caused by poor technique;
- Over-stretching of ligaments caused by poor technique or forcing at the end of the range;
- Straining other body areas due to incorrect positioning;
- Raising blood pressure caused by incorrect breathing.

Summary and aid to learning

Flexibility:

This refers to the range of movement possible at a joint.

The factors which affect flexibility are:

Joint structure: this includes the shape of the bones; the suppleness of the capsule, muscles, ligaments and tendons surrounding the joint.

Age: flexibility decreases with ageing unless it is maintained through training.

Training: flexibility will improve for all age groups following flexibility training.

Sex/gender: it is generally thought that females have greater potential for flexibility than males.

Body temperature: tissues are more flexible when they are warm.

Strength training: some strength training routines limit flexibility but generally flexibility is not affected.

Flexibility can be *maintained* through outer and full range movements.

Flexibility can be *increased* only through a programme of over stretching.

Muscles must be warmed before being stretched – **do not stretch cold muscles**.

Perform warm-up before stretch.

Methods of stretching

Ballistic: these involve bouncing or jerking at the end of the range. The final position is not held. They are not recommended as they pull against the protective reflex contraction of the muscle. This can result in microtears of muscle fibres.

Dynamic: these involve moving the muscle through short range movements and increasing to full range. The final position is momentarily held. The movements used generally copy the joint movements used in performance.

Static: these involve taking the muscle slowly to the end of full range, holding, then applying further stretch and holding the new position. This is the safest and most popular form of stretching.

Proprioceptive neuromuscular facilitation (PNF): this is also known as the *contract relax method.* One method involves performing a maximum isometric contraction against resistance at the end of the range, then relaxing the muscle and moving it further to increase the range.

Technique of static stretching

Select a warm venue and wear warm clothing.

Perform movements of large muscle groups to ensure that the tissues are thoroughly warmed.

Relax and concentrate on the muscle to be stretched.

Place the joint in the correct position.

Stretch slowly and evenly; feel the stretch in the belly of the muscle.

Hold for 6–10 seconds; this can increase to 20 seconds with practice.

As tension decreases stretch a little further and hold for 20–30 seconds.

Do not bounce or jerk at the end of range.

Move slowly out of stretch.

List three signs which indicate that you should ease out of stretch and relax.

Stretching should be performed after warm-up but before performance to increase flexibility which reduces the risk of injury.

Stretching performed after performance during cool-down, reduces muscle soreness.

QUESTIONS
1. Explain what is meant by 'the flexibility' of a joint.
2. Give three reasons why flexibility is important to an athlete.
3. Briefly explain the six factors which influence flexibility.
4. Give the two ranges of movement through which a joint must be exercised to maintain and improve flexibility.
5. Explain three reasons why ballistic stretching is not recommended.
6. Explain the following terms:
   a active stretching
   b active assisted stretching
   c passive stretching
7. List six effects of stretch training.
8. State where 'the pull' should be felt during static stretching.
9. Explain when the stretching phase should be performed within a training programme.
10. Explain why stretching should be performed before performance and after performance.

STRETCHING EXERCISES

Stretching the foot

Starting position	Exercise
■ Sitting, legs crossed at knee	gently and evenly pull the toes upwards and then the foot. Hold and relax.
■ Sitting, legs crossed at knee	gently and evenly push the foot downwards and then the toes. Hold and relax.
■ Heel sitting	with bare feet, sit back on the heels and feel the pull on the top of the foot. Hold and relax. (Caution: not to be performed by anyone with knee problems.)
■ Standing	place the toes vertically against a step, rock forwards and raise the heels off the ground.

Calf stretching

GASTROCNEMIUS AND SOLEUS

Starting position	Exercise
■ Long sitting, back against wall	keep the knees straight and strongly dorsi-flex the feet (do not invert or evert). Hold for a count of ten and release. (A strap can be placed around the balls of the feet and pulled towards the body for additional stretch.)

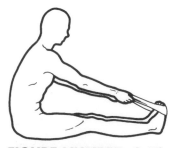

FIGURE NUMBER: 9.49

■ Walk standing, one foot directly in front of the other

keep the back heel firmly on the ground and bend the front knee gently until a pull is felt in the calf of the hind leg. Hold for a count of ten, then slowly release. Repeat with the other leg.

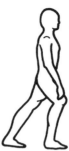

FIGURE NUMBER: 9.50

■ Reach standing, facing a wall, with hands against wall

walk the feet backwards, keeping the heels on the ground, until a pull is felt in the calves. Hold for a count of ten.

■ Standing with hands against wall as above

walk the feet backwards, keeping the heels on the ground. When the pull is just being felt, bend the elbows slowly and the pull will increase. Hold for a count of ten.

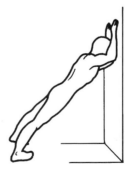

FIGURE NUMBER: 9.51

■ Standing on an incline

lean forward, keeping the heels on the ground, until a pull is felt in the calf.

■ Toe standing on the edge of a step

lift up onto the toes and align the body over the feet, then lower the heels until the pull is felt in the calf. Hold for a count of ten, then release.

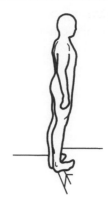

FIGURE NUMBER: 9.52

- Reach standing, hands against wall

keeping the heels on the ground bend both knees, then take the body forward over the feet until the pull is felt in the calf. Hold for a count of ten, then release.

Front of thigh stretching

QUADRICEPS GROUP: RECTUS FEMORIS, VASTUS MEDIALIS, VASTUS LATERALIS AND VASTUS INTERMEDIUS

Starting position	*Exercise*
■ Support standing	standing on one leg, grasp the other leg from behind around the ankle. Pull the leg backwards until the pull is felt in the front of the thigh. Hold for a count of ten, then release. Keep the trunk straight and avoid rotating the hip and knee outwards. Repeat with the other leg.

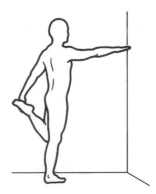

FIGURE NUMBER: 9.53

■ Prone lying

bend the right knee towards the buttock, grasp the ankle and pull until the pull is felt in the front of the thigh. Hold for a count of ten, then release. Keep the front of the hip joint against the floor. Repeat with the other leg.

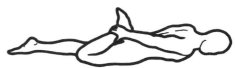

FIGURE NUMBER: 9.54

Fit individuals with no back problems can repeat the above exercise with both knees bent, pulling on both ankles together.

■ Side lying

bending one leg, pull the heel towards the buttocks. Repeat with the other leg.

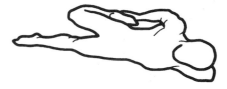

FIGURE NUMBER: 9.55

■ Kneeling

lean backwards, keeping the hips pushed forward, until a pull is felt in front of thigh. Hold for a count of ten, then sit forward. (Caution: not for older clients or anyone with knee problems.)

Back of thigh stretching

HAMSTRINGS: BICEPS FEMORIS, SEMIMEMBRANOSUS, SEMITENDINOSUS

Starting position	Exercise
■ Supine lying with hips and knees at right angles and feet against a wall	slide the right leg up the wall, dorsi-flex the foot and tighten the knee. Keeping the leg straight and the bottom on the floor, lift the leg away from the wall. Hold for a count of ten and place the foot back on the wall. Repeat with the other leg.
■ Crook lying	lift the right leg up and clasp the hands behind the knee. Straighten the knee and dorsi-flex the foot until the pull is felt in the back of the thigh. Hold for a count of ten and lower back to crook. Repeat with the other leg. (Caution: stop if the back arches.)

FIGURE NUMBER: 9.56

■ Standing in front of a stool or stairs	place one leg onto the stool or the second step of the stairs. Reach forward towards the foot, keeping the back straight and the head in line. Move forward until the pull is felt in the back of the thigh. Hold for a count of ten and release. Repeat with the other leg.
■ Modified Hurdler's stretch	bend other leg and place foot against inner thigh. Roll knees out slightly. With straight back and head in line, lean over straight leg until pull is felt in back of the thigh.

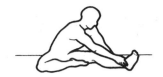

FIGURE NUMBER: 9.57

Inner thigh stretching

ADDUCTOR GROUP: ADDUCTOR LONGUS, ADDUCTOR MAGNUS, ADDUCTOR BREVIS, PECTINEUS, GRACILIS

Starting position	Exercise
■ Long sitting	open the legs as far as possible. Keep the back straight and lean forwards until a pull is felt in the inner thigh. Hold for a count of ten and release. (Caution: do not round the trunk or slouch.)
■ Crook sitting	keep the feet together and drop the knees open as far as possible. Then pull the feet towards the body until the pull is felt in the inner thigh. Hold for a count of ten and release. (Caution: not to be done by anyone with knee or hip problems.)

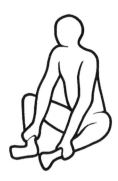

FIGURE NUMBER: 9.58

■ Crook lying, hands on knees

part the knees as far as possible, then press apart with the hands until the pull is felt on the inside of the thigh. Hold for a count of ten and release. (Caution: not to be done by anyone with knee or hip problems.)

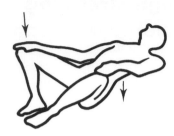

FIGURE NUMBER: 9.59

■ Supine lying, legs up against a wall

part the legs by sliding them along the wall until a stretch is felt in the inner thigh. Hold for a count of ten and release.

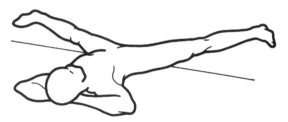

FIGURE NUMBER: 9.60

■ Stride standing

stretch the right leg out as far sideways as possible, without rotating the leg outwards, then bend the left leg until a pull is felt on inner thigh of the right leg. Hold for a count of ten and release. Repeat with the other leg.

Outer thigh stretching

HIP ABDUCTORS: GLUTEUS MEDIUS, GLUTEUS MINIMUS, TENSOR FASCIA LATA

Starting position	Exercise
▪ Supine lying	raise the right leg and swing it over the left leg. Lift the right leg slightly and dorsi-flex the foot until a pull is felt at the outer thigh. Hold for a count of ten, then release. Repeat with the other leg.

FIGURE NUMBER: 9.61

Starting position	Exercise
▪ Supine lying	bend the left knee to the chest, then push the knee across to the right until a pull is felt in the outer thigh. Hold for a count of ten and release. Repeat with the other leg.

FIGURE NUMBER: 9.62

Starting position	Exercise
▪ Supine lying	raise the leg to vertical and move it across the body until a pull is felt in the outer thigh. Repeat with the other leg.

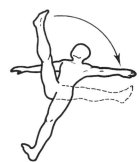

FIGURE NUMBER: 9.63

- Standing

take the right leg across behind the left as far as possible and place the foot on the ground with the toes turned in. Take the body weight through this leg until a pull is felt in the outer thigh. Hold for a count of ten, then release. Repeat with the other leg.

- Long sitting

bend the right knee and place the foot on the far side of the left leg, level with the knee. Push the bent knee over the left until a pull is felt in the outer thigh. Hold for a count of ten and release. Repeat with the other leg.

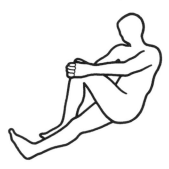

FIGURE NUMBER: 9.64

Buttock stretching

HIP EXTENSORS: GLUTEUS MAXIMUS

Starting position	Exercise
■ Lying	bend the right knee onto the chest, then pull the knee closer, keeping the other leg straight and the back flat against the floor until a pull is felt in the buttock. Hold for a count of ten and release. Repeat with the other leg.

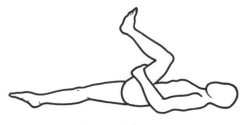

FIGURE NUMBER: 9.65

▣ Inclined prone kneeling	stretch the hands forwards onto the floor, bend the right knee towards the hands, then drop the trunk onto the thigh. Hold for a count of ten and release. Repeat with the other leg. (Caution: not to be done by anyone with knee problems.)
▣ Standing	bend the right knee to the chest then pull the knee closer, but do not arch the back. Hold for a count of ten and release. Repeat with the other leg.
▣ Standing	place the right foot on a step, then drop the trunk forward and inside the leg, bending the left knee until a pull is felt in the right buttock. Hold for a count of ten and release. Repeat with the other leg.
▣ Crook lying	bend the right leg up and place the ankle across the left thigh. Lift the left leg up and back to apply pressure on the right leg until a pull is felt in the right buttock. Hold for a count of ten and release. Repeat with the other leg.

Hip flexor stretching

PSOAS AND ILIACUS, SARTORIUS

Starting position	Exercise
▣ Walk standing	bend the forward knee, feeling the pull in the other hip. Repeat with the other leg.

FIGURE NUMBER: 9.66

■ Supine lying

press one leg firmly against the floor and bend the other leg onto the chest. Pull the bent leg with the hands, feeling the pull in front of the hip on the straight leg. Hold and release. Repeat with the other leg.

■ Half kneeling

lean forwards over the bent knee and feel the pull in the other hip. Hold and release. Repeat with the other leg.

FIGURE NUMBER: 9.67

■ Prone kneeling

lift one leg up behind and place it on a chair with the knee supported. Bend the other knee and let the body move downwards, feeling the stretch on the straight leg. Hold and release. Repeat with the other leg.

■ Crook lying

lift the buttocks off the floor, pushing upwards as high as possible. Hold and release.

Lower back stretching

ERECTOR SPINAE AND QUADRATUS LUMBORUM

Starting position	Exercise
■ Crook lying	pressing the small of the back into the floor, bring the right knee onto the chest. Clasp the hands around the knee and pull it towards the chest. Hold then relax. Repeat with the other leg.

■ Crook lying

pressing the small of the back into the floor, bring both knees onto the chest. Clasp the hands around the thighs and pull them towards the chest. Hold for a count of ten and release.

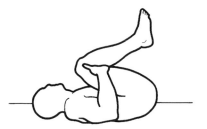

FIGURE NUMBER: 9.68

■ Crook lying

as above, but also lift the head and shoulders off the ground. Hold for a count of ten and release.

■ Crook lying

keeping the knees together, drop them down to the right, feeling a pull on left side. Hold and release. Then drop the knees to the other side. Hold and release.

■ Yard lying

bend the right knee and place the foot outside the left knee. Bring the left hand down and pull the knee to the left, keeping the right arm and shoulder on the floor. Hold and release. Repeat with the other leg.

FIGURE NUMBER: 9.69

■ Prone kneeling

contract the abdominals and round the back, then lower it to horizontal.

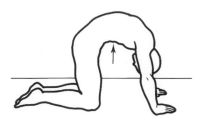

FIGURE NUMBER: 9.70

■ Crook lying with a firm rolled towel under the sacrum

press the lower back against the floor. Hold and release.

■ Sitting with feet on floor

lean the body forward, taking the trunk down to the thighs. Hang the arms at the sides.

Arm stretching

BICEPS, TRICEPS, LATISSIMUS DORSI

Starting position	Exercise
■ Stride standing	*Biceps stretch* clasp the hands behind the back. Keeping the elbows straight, raise the arms upwards. Hold for a count of ten and release.

FIGURE NUMBER: 9.71

■ Stride standing

lift a bar above the head and stretch the arms backwards. Keep the elbows straight.

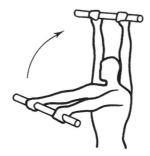

FIGURE NUMBER: 9.72

■ Stride standing

Triceps stretch
lift the right arm upwards and
bend the elbow so that the hand
lies behind the head. Use the
other hand behind the head to
push the upper arm down further.
Repeat with the other arm.

■ Stride standing

clasp the hands above the head,
and pull the arms backwards as far
as possible behind the head. Hold
for a count of ten and release.

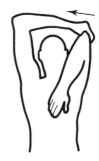

FIGURE NUMBER: 9.73

■ Sitting

Latissimus dorsi stretch
Lift one arm upwards and bend
the elbow so that the hand lies
behind the head. Use the other
hand to pull the arm towards the
body and bend the trunk to the
same side. Hold and release.
Repeat with the other arm.
(Caution do not side Flex Trunk. Bend
only until pull is felt below armpit. Only
suitable for young or agile.)

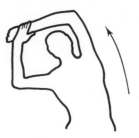

FIGURE NUMBER: 9.74

■ Stretch stride standing

place the backs of the hands together and stretch towards the ceiling.

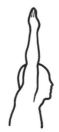

FIGURE NUMBER: 9.75

Front of thorax stretching

PECTORALIS MAJOR

Starting position	Exercise
■ Stride standing	press the shoulders backwards.
■ Crook lying, arms at sides	place a tightly rolled hand towel lengthways between the scapulae. Press the shoulders down into the floor.
■ Crook lying, arms out to side, elbows at right angles, palms facing upwards	the same action as above.
■ Yard crook lying	the same action as above.

FIGURE NUMBER: 9.76

■ Prone kneeling

stretch the arms forwards and outwards until the elbows are straight. Extend the wrists and drop the chest forwards, pulling the shoulders backwards.

■ Lying with a pillow between the shoulders

raise the arms above the head and press them into the floor.

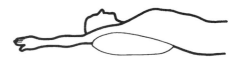

FIGURE NUMBER: 9.77

■ Stride standing or high sitting

place one bent arm behind the head with the elbow pointing upwards, the other behind the back with the elbow pointing downwards. Clasp the hands if possible, or link them with a towel or strap. Pull downwards, bringing the upper arm back and nearer the head. Repeat with the other arm.

■ Stride standing or high sitting

use a bar that is shoulder-width long or just over. Hold the bar at the ends, lift it upwards above the head and then lower it downwards behind the head.

■ Long sitting with back to a chair or wall bars

place the arms behind and grasp the sides of the chair. Keep the elbows straight and thrust the chest upwards and forwards, keeping the chin in. Hold then release.

■ Standing with back to wall bars

place the arms behind and grasp the wall bar just below shoulder height. Drop the body forward and pull back between the scapulae. Keep the chin in. Hold and release.

■ Walk standing in an open doorway

with the elbows and shoulders at right angles, place one hand on the wall on either side of the doorway. Lean forward into the doorway.

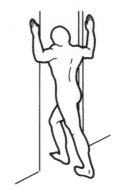

FIGURE NUMBER: 9.78

TASKS

■ Devise exercise schemes for stretching the following muscles – gastrocnemius; quadriceps; hamstrings; hip flexors; back extensors; pectorals.

■ Teach one of your schemes to a partner or group.

SPEED

Speed is the distance moved in a specific time:

$$\text{Speed} = \frac{\text{distance moved}}{\text{time taken}}$$

Speed is a requirement of many activities in athletics and sport. Speed may be required in the lower limbs for sprinting, in the upper limbs for throwing or fast bowling or in both for certain sports such as basketball. Speed is related to muscle strength, flexibility, reaction time and leverage.

Strength

Muscle force is necessary to produce acceleration. The greater the force applied by the muscles, the greater the acceleration and speed. In sprinting, the push-off muscles of the propelling leg will drive the body forward. The greater the strength of these muscles, the greater the driving force. These muscles are the gastrocnemius and soleus in the calf, the quadriceps on the front of the thigh and the gluteus maximus in the buttock. Strengthening exercises for these muscles should form part of the training regime to increase speed. For throwing speed, strengthening exercises are required for the serratus anterior, pectoralis major, anterior deltoid, triceps, wrist and finger extensors.

Flexibility

A large range of movement at the joints will allow for longer strides, and long fast strides will increase speed. Increased flexibility of the ankle, knee and hip will thus increase running speed. Increased flexibility of the shoulder, elbow and wrist will increase the propulsion force when throwing. Flexibility exercises should therefore be included in training programmes.

Reaction time

The ability to react quickly to a stimulus is vital in many sports. Muscles must be able to contract instantly in response to a stimulus such as a starting gun or the hitting of a service ball. Instant reactions to stimuli will improve speed. Reaction time can be improved by repetitive practice of the required action, optimising body position and nervous response. Exercises where a quick response is required, such as ball throwing, catching and running, are also used.

Leverage

Body activities involve the movement of many levers. As previously explained (chapter 7), the levers of the human body are mainly of the third order. These are designed for speed and range of movement. The longer the lever, the greater the speed, providing the force or muscle strength is great enough.

The effect of lactic acid on speed

The build-up of lactic acid has an inhibitory effect on muscle contraction. Bursts of fast activity initially use stored ATP and PC, but these are soon used up and fast energy is obtained from the anaerobic breakdown of glycogen into pyruvic acid with the production of lactic acid. This build-up of lactic acid inhibits muscle contraction and therefore reduces speed. Athletes must therefore train to increase their aerobic capacity and to run close to their VO_2max. Since the aerobic metabolism is used for a longer period, there will be little or no lactic acid and little impairment of the muscle action.

This form of training will consist initially of short bursts of intense activity for 30–60 seconds and then rests of the same duration. The time is then progressively increased. These activities may include shuttle running or a circuit of set exercises interspersed with running. Training for speed involves different forms of running, beginning with jogging, moving on to running and finishing with maximum-speed sprinting. Variations include maximum-pace running interspersed with walking or jogging. Training must also include specific training at maximum speed for set distances.

Other physical principles affecting speed include reaction forces, friction, resistance forces and mass.

SKILL

Skilled movement is balanced, co-ordinated, graceful and precise, with accurate timing and overall rhythmic flow. There is no wastage of energy.

Skill is learnt behaviour and improves as a result of practice and experience. Acquiring a skill is goal-directed: the learner must be aware of the desired end result and how to achieve it. Constant repetitions of patterns of movement must be practised until they are registered in the brain and can eventually be performed automatically (see chapter 12). In order to master an activity and give a skilled performance, the activity should be broken down into small chunks or parts. Each part should be practised until a satisfactory standard is achieved. The sequence of movements is then linked, and the complete activity is practised until all errors are eliminated and the performance is automatic. Muscle strength and flexibility contribute to a skilled performance, but other factors are involved, such as neuro-muscular co-ordination, balance, etc.

Balance will improve by gradually reducing stability. Practice of a movement should begin in a stable position and progress to a less stable position. The speed of performance can also vary from normal to slow and then fast. Rhythm and timing will improve as the activity is mastered and co-ordination, grace and precision are achieved.

Summary and aid to learning

Speed is the distance moved in a specific time.

Speed times strength equals power.

Speed is a requirement of many sports and contributes to maximum performance.

List six sporting or athletic activities where you think speed is important.

The factors which influence speed are:
strength – greater strength means greater driving force or propulsion; *flexibility* – greater flexibility means greater range of movement, longer strides, etc.; *reaction time* – the faster the response to a stimulus or instant reaction will improve speed; *leverage* – long levers improve speed; lactic acid build up – because the build up of lactic acid inhibits muscle contraction speed will be reduced.

Motor skill is precision of movement with no wastage of energy.

Skill is learnt behaviour and goal directed.

Factors which contribute to motor skill are:
strength, flexibility, neuro-muscular coordination, balance, rhythm, etc.

Skill is an area of study which is not within the scope of this book.

NUTRITION AND DIET

This is a vast and specialised field, the detail of which is not within the scope of this book. Therapists requiring detailed information should therefore refer to specialist texts. However, this chapter should provide you with a solid foundation for this important topic.

The food we eat is broken down by the digestive system and used to maintain body functions such as:

- providing energy for cellular activity;
- providing building material for tissue growth and repair;
- producing hormones, enzymes and antibodies.

A good balanced diet must be eaten to supply all the nutrients necessary for the body to perform its functions and promote health. Any food which is surplus to requirements is converted into fat and stored in adipose tissue. These fat stores are our fuel storage tanks; in times of high demand or low calorie intake, this fat is removed and broken down to provide energy for muscle contraction and cellular activity.

Energy

Energy may be defined as the capacity to perform work. The energy requirements of the body will vary depending on the activities carried out. The basic energy requirement of the body for maintaining body functions in the waking state is known as the *basal metabolic rate* (BMR). This refers to the condition of the body first thing in the morning before getting up, or after lying down for at least 60 minutes. BMR is proportional to body weight: the heavier you are, the higher your BMR will be. It is generally higher for men and decreases with age. The demand for energy will proportionally increase as body activities increase, i.e. the greater the intensity of the activity, the greater the energy expenditure will be.

Calories

A calorie is a unit of heat used to express the energy value of food.

- A calorie is the heat required to raise the temperature of one gram of water by 1 degree Celsius.
- A Kilocalorie (Kcal) is the heat required to raise one Kilogram of water by 1 degree Celsius.

The metric measurement of the energy value of food is the kilojoule. To convert Kcal to KJ: 1 Kcal = 4.2 KJ

Calorie intake should never be below one's basal metabolic rate; low calorie diets of 1,000 Kcals or below are dangerous. A well-balanced diet of around 1,500 Kcals per day should provide adequate nutrients for those leading sedentary lives, but most people require more. The average active female consumes over 2,000 Kcals per day and the average male consumes over 3,000

Kcals. However, for anyone involved in intense physical activity, e.g. athletes, sports people etc., this will rise to 4,000–6,000 Kcals and above. These individuals must carefully consider their diet to ensure that they are meeting their energy demands.

Essential nutrients

There are six basic nutrients necessary for a healthy diet:

- carbohydrates
- fats (lipids)
- proteins
- vitamins
- minerals
- water.

Fibre is an additional requirement, as it aids the functioning of the digestive tract and protects against many diseases.

Carbohydrates, fats and proteins are the energy providers and are known as *energy nutrients* or *macronutrients*. The other nutrients play important roles but they do not provide energy; they are known as *micronutrients*. Other chemical compounds derived from plants known as *phyto chemicals* have recently been identified which offer protection against carcinogens (substances which produce cancer).

Carbohydrates

Carbohydrates give the body its source of quick energy, and are the starches, sugars and cellulose found in pulses, cereals, bread, honey, potatoes, pasta, rice, and root vegetables. They are composed of carbon, hydrogen, and oxygen.

Carbohydrates are divided into three main groups:

1 Monosaccharides (glucose, fructose and galactose);
2 Dissaccharides (sucrose, lactose and maltose);
3 Polysaccharides (starches, glycogen, and cellulose).

During digestion, complex sugars (polysaccharides) are broken down to simple sugars (disaccharides) and then to one unit sugars (monosaccharides). These are absorbed in the small intestine and transported in the blood to the liver, where fructose and galactose are converted to glucose.

Sources of carbohydrate in our diet

Simple carbohydrates (monosaccharides and disaccharides) are the sugars found in honey, syrups, jams or fruits, etc. They give a quick surge of energy which quickly disappears, making us feel tired and craving for more. Sugar and refined carbohydrates (white flour, white rice, etc.) are low in vitamins, minerals and fibre and are therefore not as nutritious as unrefined and complex carbohydrates.

Complex carbohydrates (polysaccharides) are starches and fibre. They are found in bread, cakes, pasta, cereals, pulses, fruit and vegetables. They should form the greater percentage of our dietary intake because they provide vitamins, minerals, fibre and phyto chemicals. *Unrefined*, wholemeal products (e.g. brown rice, wholemeal bread and pasta) have a high nutritional value.

Glucose

Glucose obtained from the breakdown of carbohydrates is used to produce ATP (adenosine tri-phosphate) required for muscle contraction. After eating a meal, blood sugar (glucose) levels will rise, which stimulates the pancreas to secrete insulin. Insulin reduces blood sugar levels, as it aids the transport of glucose from the blood into the cells. Glucose is then either used directly by the cells for immediate energy, or is converted in the liver to glycogen by a process known as *glycogenesis*. This glycogen is then stored in the liver or in muscle tissue, and will provide a reserve of energy for future use. When these stores are full, surplus glucose is converted in the liver to fat, which is then stored as triglycerides in adipose tissue. Thus, a low fat but high carbohydrate diet may still increase body fat if all the carbohydrate is not utilised for energy. When energy demands are high, stored glycogen is needed. The liver then converts glycogen back to glucose, to supply the energy required. This process is known as *glycogenolysis*.

> **LEARN**
> One gram of carbohydrate yields approximately 4.0 Kcals of energy

The body is only able to store a small amount of glycogen – around 500 g – which amounts to around 2000 Kcals of energy. Of this, approximately 80 percent is stored in skeletal muscle tissue and 20% in the liver. This is only enough to provide energy for one day of normal activity, so a regular intake of carbohydrate is necessary to maintain glycogen stores.

The average person with a sedentary life style should derive over 50 percent of total daily calories from carbohydrates (this means consuming over 300 g daily). The athlete or anyone with high energy expenditure will require over 60–70 percent which means over 400–600 g daily.

The use of carbohydrates during exercise

Glycogen will be used to produce ATP during all forms of exercise, but the proportion used increases with the intensity and decreases with the duration of the activity. During short bursts of intense anaerobic activity, such as fast short duration sprints, stored ATP, phosphocreatine and glycogen provide the energy. During prolonged moderate or intense aerobic activity, carbohydrates will be the main source, but a proportion will be supplied by fats. Prolonged low intensity activity such as distance walking or jogging will use a greater percentage of fat.

Following any intense activity, muscle and liver glycogen will be depleted. It is important to restore glycogen levels as quickly as possible after exercise, by eating a high carbohydrate meal. The more depleted the store, the longer it will take to restore and the more carbohydrate will be required. It is recommended that 1 g of carbohydrate is eaten for every kilogram of body weight.

Exercising with low glycogen levels will lead to early muscle fatigue and poor performance. It is therefore vital for athletes, sports people, etc., to ensure a high carbohydrate intake as this will enable them to exercise for longer and to improve performance.

Research has shown that a high carbohydrate diet significantly increases endurance. Long distance runners increase carbohydrate intake to around 80 percent of total calorie intake to enhance performance. These athletes may practise the technique of *carbohydrate loading*, to substantially increase glycogen stores. This involves depleting glycogen stores for three days through exercise and diet, followed by a high consumption of carbohydrates two to three days before the event. However, this is no longer recommended, and at most should only be done twice or three times a year, as it can lead to fatigue and health risks. Different techniques of carbohydrate loading are being introduced, including gradually decreasing the duration of training and increasing carbohydrate intake for seven days before performance.

During any activity of 60 minutes or over, carbohydrate intake can help to delay fatigue. Suitable consumables include carbohydrate sports drinks, or a banana.

Fats

Fats are the body's secondary source of energy: carbohydrates provide primary fast energy, while fats provide long-term energy. Like carbohydrates, they are composed of carbon, hydrogen, and oxygen but in a different ratio – there is less oxygen in fats. Fats or lipids are obtained from animal and vegetable sources.

Sources of fat in our diet

There are two main types of fat:

- saturated
- unsaturated.

Saturated fats

These contain the maximum number of hydrogen atoms in each molecule, and so are *saturated* with respect to hydrogen. They tend to be solid at room temperature. Saturated fats are found mainly in animal products such as pork, beef, lamb, butter, milk, cheese, eggs, etc. They are also found in certain plant products such as cocoa butter, palm oil and coconut oil. These fats contribute to high blood cholesterol levels and heart disease, and their excessive consumption should be discouraged.

Unsaturated fats

These contain fewer hydrogen atoms, and so are called *unsaturated*. This group include monounsaturated fats and polyunsaturated fats. These come mainly from plant sources, and tend to be liquid at room temperature.

- Monounsaturates include olive oil and peanut oil.
- Polyunsaturates include corn oil, sunflower oil, sesame oil, cotton seed oil, soybean oil.

These fats help to reduce cholesterol levels; the consumption of these fats, in particular the monosaturates, is preferable to saturated fats.

The use of fats during exercise

Both saturated and unsaturated fats provide the same amount of energy per unit weight:

> **LEARN**
> One gram of fat yields approximately 9.0 Kcals of energy

In addition to providing energy, fats protect vital organs such as the heart and kidneys, they provide body insulation, and are used in many physiological processes such as resynthesising tissues e.g. the myelin sheaths of nerves and thromboplastin for blood clotting. They also transport the fat soluble vitamins.

During digestion, fats are broken down to fatty acids and glycerol. If these fatty acids are not required for immediate energy, they are converted and stored in adipose tissue and in the liver in the form of triglycerides.

Fats are the body's most concentrated source of energy. Twice as much energy is stored in one gram of fat, than in one gram of carbohydrate. The body is able to store far more fat than glycogen, and so it is a greater store of potential energy which allows us to exercise for very long periods; even marathon runners do not run out of fat. However, fat requires a small amount of glycogen for its combustion and if glycogen stores are depleted, fat cannot be broken down to provide energy.

Fat cannot provide energy for fast activity, because it depends on the availability of oxygen, which depends on a person's aerobic capacity. A fit person with high aerobic capacity will burn fat more easily than an unfit person. During medium pace activities, fat provides around 50 percent of the required energy. If the effort is prolonged, fat will provide up to 90 percent of the required energy.

High fat intake increases the likelihood of developing high cholesterol levels, hypertension and heart diseases. It is also linked with the development of many cancers, such as breast and colon cancers. It is recommended that fat intake should not exceed 20–30 percent of total energy intake; of this only 6–10 percent should be saturated fat.

Cholesterol

Cholesterol is a fatty like substance belonging to the chemical group known as *sterols*. Cholesterol is consumed in the diet, but is also synthesised in the liver. A high intake of saturated fat increases cholesterol levels, but it is also found in red meats, liver, kidney, egg yolk and dairy products. (It is not found in vegetables.) A certain amount of cholesterol is needed by the body for building cells and producing hormones, but too much is harmful, as it contributes to plaque formation in the arteries, which causes blockages and clots and increases the risk of coronary heart disease. Cholesterol is bound to two types of lipoproteins:

1 high density lipoproteins (HDL) – this is 'good' cholesterol as it does not adhere to vessel walls and may even protect against heart disease.
2 low density lipoproteins (LDL) – this is the 'bad' high risk cholesterol.

A low intake of saturated fats and cholestrol rich foods is recommended to protect against heart disease.

Proteins

Proteins are chemically different from carbohydrates and fats, and are more complex in structure. They are composed of carbon, hydrogen and oxygen, but also contain nitrogen, sulphur and iron.

Proteins are the tissue builders of the body, used for growth, body building and tissue repair. Proteins are:

- used in the growth and repair of keratin, collagen, elastin
- used in the production of actin and myosin, which increase the size of myofibrils and the strength of muscle contraction.
- needed to repair damage following injuries such as bone fractures, muscle strains, tendon and ligamentous injuries etc.
- essential in rebuilding muscle cells after intense effort
- catalysts for many chemical reactions
- thought to have an effect on the nervous system, increasing arousal and alertness, which are important for the elite performer
- used for making antibodies, enzymes and hormones.

Proteins are constructed from amino acids. There are 20 amino acids required by the body, and most can be manufactured by the body. However, eight cannot, and must be taken in from the diet; and these are known as *essential amino acids*.

Proteins are manufactured in the cells of plants and animals. Those containing all the essential amino acids are called *complete proteins* (high quality proteins). These are generally obtained from animal sources such as lean meat, fish, eggs, milk and cheese. Those which do not contain all the essential amino acids are called *incomplete proteins* (low quality), which are obtained from plant sources such as grains, pulses, fruit and vegetables. Vegans and vegetarians must ensure that they eat a wide variety of these products, to ensure an adequate intake of essential amino acids.

Food containing protein is broken down by the digestive system into amino acids. Those taken directly into cells are synthesised into new proteins, and the remainder are taken to the liver where some are synthesised into plasma proteins, others are de-animated and used for energy if required, or converted to glycogen or fat and stored.

There are no protein stores in the body, unlike carbohydrate and fat stores. All body protein is functional, therefore the body must ingest enough protein to meet its needs. Protein intake should be 10–15 percent of total energy intake i.e. 70–100 g per day. This should increase in times of illness, growth, tissue repair, during pregnancy or training and performance. Many elite performers increase their protein intake with supplements of amino acids (but there is no evidence to date to prove that taking supplements enhances performance).

> **LEARN**
> One gram of protein yields 4.0 Kcals of energy

Proteins are only used as an energy source in cases of starvation, or very long distance running when all stores of carbohydrates and fats are running low.

Vitamins

Vitamins are chemical compounds. They are essential nutrients which enable the body to function efficiently, but they do not provide energy. They do, however, play important roles:

- they regulate metabolic processes;
- they are important for growth, for the functioning of the nervous system and the immune system;
- they are involved in enzyme production, and in many other biological functions.

Vitamins are obtained from plant and animals food sources, and a balanced diet will ensure an adequate intake. Vitamins K and B_6 are formed by bacterial action in the large intestine, but the others must be obtained from the diet.

Vitamins may be grouped into:
- Fat soluble vitamins (A, D, E, K)
- Water soluble vitamins (B complex and C)

Fat soluble vitamins are stored in the liver and in fatty tissue whereas water soluble vitamins are excreted in the urine.

Fat soluble vitamins

Vitamin A
Source: fish oils, butter, milk, cheese, eggs. Our body can produce this vitamin from *carotenoids*, e.g. beta-carotene found in yellow vegetables and fruits such as carrots, peaches, apricots, melon and in green leafy vegetables such as spinach and broccoli.
Function: aids growth and repair of tissues; maintains mucous membranes, epithelial linings, and skin. Provides a visual pigment required for night vision. Beta-carotene may protect against heart attack, cancer, and reduce muscle soreness.
Deficiency: nightblindness.

Vitamin D
Source: fish oils, eggs, dairy products, fortified cereals, margarines. Produced in the skin by the action of sunlight on dehydrocholesterol.
Function: increases the absorption of calcium; promotes the growth of bones.
Deficiency: rickets, brittle bones and bone deformities.

Vitamin E
Source: Wheatgerm, wholemeal cereals and bread, nuts, seeds, egg yolk, vegetable oils.
Function: As an antioxidant it helps to protect against cancer, heart disease; it protects cell membranes; it helps muscles to utilise oxygen and may aid recovery after exercise.
Deficiency: possibly anaemia.

Vitamin K
Source: green vegetables, fruits, cereals, meat.
Function: involved in the formation or prothrombin; essential in blood clotting.
Deficiency: increased risk of haemorrhages.

Water soluble vitamins

Vitamin B complex
This is a large group of vitamins; each has a particular function.
Source: obtained from a wide variety of sources: lean meats, vegetables, pulses, legumes, whole grains, dairy products, eggs.
Function: They are essential for:

- creating energy;
- converting carbohydrates into glucose;
- the metabolism of fats and proteins.

Some are associated with the manufacture of red blood cells, the growth and development of cells, and with the functioning of the nervous system.
Deficiency: as this group of vitamins has a wide range of functions, deficiency will result in many disorders and conditions – beriberi, pellagra, fatigue, muscular twitching, anaemia, nervous disorders, gastrointestinal problems.
Folic acid: this is included in the B vitamins. It helps to form heme, the iron containing protein which is needed to form red blood cells. It protects coronary vessels and is required for brain development and function.

Vitamin C
Source: citrus fruits, berries, tomatoes, peppers, leafy green vegetables.
Functions: growth and tissue repair; collagen formation; important for healthy gums, teeth and blood vessels; it helps to absorb iron and utilise folic acid; it forms adrenaline; it helps fight bacteria, is an antioxidant and may help fight cancer.
Deficiency: scurvy, anaemia, poor connective tissue growth and repair, tender swollen gums and loose teeth, bleeding, decrease in exercise performance as it affects aerobic capacity.

Minerals

Minerals are found in all body cells and fluids, and they form part of the body's structure. Although these elements are only required in small quantities, they are esential for regulating and maintaining life processes. They cannot be manufactured by the body and must be obtained from the diet.

Calcium

Calcium is required for the formation of teeth and bones. Inadequate intake of calcium results in porous bones, known as *osteoporosis*. Menopausal women are particularly susceptible to this disease, as there is a loss of bone mass and a high risk of sustaining bone fractures. Regular exercise, an active lifestyle and an adequate calcium intake will protect against this disease.

Iron is an important mineral, as it is a component of haemoglobin and muscle myoglobin. An adequate iron intake is therefore important for transportation and the storage of oxygen. Female athletes in particular must guard against iron deficiency (anaemia), as this will affect aerobic capacity.

Other minerals such as **sodium**, **potassium** and **magnesium** are important for nerve impulse conduction and fluid balance. **Iodine** is required for proper functioning of the thyroid gland.

Profuse sweating will result in water and mineral loss which must be replaced through a balanced diet. Sports drinks can help in cases of severe fluid loss.

Vitamin and mineral requirements of the athlete

Manufacturers imply that the athlete will derive great benefit from taking vitamin and mineral supplements. These micronutrients do *not* provide energy, and research indicates that there is no benefit in consuming extra vitamins if recommended levels are maintained through a varied and balanced diet. It is true that these nutrients are essential for the proper functioning of bodily processes but they are only required in small amounts.

Nutritional requirements will vary depending on age, size, levels of activity and metabolism. Individuals who are very active will require more than those who are inactive, but because they generally eat more, they will obtain an adequate supply of nutrients naturally from food. Supplements may be advisable for those who are restricting calories or for vegans; they may also be recommended following illness, during pregnancy, or for those suffering from anaemia or other deficiency diseases.

Performance may be adversely affected if the intake of vitamins and minerals is below the recommended levels, but providing intake meets the recommended levels, performance will not be further improved by consuming large doses above this level. Advice should be sought from a doctor or qualified nutritionist before taking supplements.

When deficiency has been investigated and established, supplements must be limited to the recommended dose, and balanced to include all the nutrients which contribute in some way to performance. For example:
- vitamin A, for repair of tissues
- vitamin B complex, involved in energy metabolism

- vitamin C, necessary for the absorption of iron and the forming of red blood cells which transport oxygen
- vitamins C, E and beta-carotene to neutralise free radicals, thus limiting post exercise pain and soreness (explained below)
- calcium, for strong bones
- iron, to improve the oxygen capacity of the blood
- magnesium, for nerve-muscle function, regulation of body temperature and to activate the enzymes involved in energy production
- potassium and sodium, for nerve-muscle function
- phosphorus as part of ATP, for energy release
- zinc, for tissue growth and repair and as a part of the enzymes required for metabolism of macro-nutrients.

Chemicals which affect the body

Free radicals

Free radicals are reactive chemicals; they are unstable atoms or molecules with unpaired electrons. They are continually produced in the body as a result of metabolic reactions, and are constantly trying to pair up with other electrons to regain stability. In their effort to become stable, they bombard other cells, damaging the cells and their DNA.

They may damage skin cells causing ageing, liver spots or skin cancers; they also damage the cells of other tissues producing various types of cancer. They attack and oxidise LDL cholesterol in the blood stream, resulting in a 'furry' plaque which blocks arteries and increases the risk of heart disease. Research has shown that there is a marked rise in free radical levels following exercise, and that they may be responsible for post exercise pain and stiffness. Fortunately substances have been identified that counter the effects of free radicals, which are known as **antioxidants**.

Antioxidants

These act as scavengers, neutralising free radicals and thus protecting the body from damage. Some are found in the body as parts of enzymes, whereas others must be consumed in the diet; e.g., vitamins C, E and beta carotene, minerals such as zinc, copper, selenium and the many phyto chemicals found in fruit and vegetables. Research indicates that these phyto chemicals afford effective protection against free radicals and cancer.

Phyto chemicals

These are chemicals such as flavonoids, sulphoraphane and chlorogenic acid. They are found in fruits and plants, which, when eaten in adequate amounts, protect the body from carcinogens and promote health.

Research indicates that at least five portions of fruits and vegetables should be eaten daily. The following fruits and vegetables will provide a variety of different phyto chemical, each having different protective effects:

■ Broccoli, cauliflower, cabbage, sprouts, kale, tomatoes, peppers, pineapples, strawberries, grapes, raspberries, onion, garlic and soya beans.

In fact, most fruit and vegetables offer some form of protection.

Water and other liquids

Water represents 40–70 percent of total body mass. Individuals who are lean and muscular have a higher water content than fatter individuals with the same body mass, because fat contains less water. The body does not store water – it is excreted in urine. If water loss is high, the body will quickly become **dehydrated** and death will occur within days. Under normal conditions, the body maintains a balance between fluid intake and output; feelings of thirst indicate that the body is dehydrated and that water is needed.

Water is essential for the biological functioning of the body:
■ it plays a vital role in regulating body temperature
■ substances dissolve in water and are transported around the body in blood plasma and lymph;
■ it is a component of cells and tissue fluid and provides a medium for the exchange of oxygen, nutrients and waste products between cells and the blood;
■ as part of synovial fluid, it lubricates joints and reduces friction;
■ it bathes tissues such as the eyes, brain and spinal cord;
■ waste products are excreted in water, as urine and faeces;
■ it absorbs heat and cools the body through evaporation. Dehydration occurs quickly during vigorous activity through profuse sweating and expired air.

To maintain water balance, the average person with a sedentary lifestyle should drink between two and three litres of water or diluted fruit juices every day. This is in addition to any tea, coffee or alcohol consumed because these are diuretics, which increase fluid loss.

Although it is a very unusual occurrence, it is important to remember that drinking *too* much water (over nine to ten litres per day) is dangerous. This will produce symptoms such as headache, blurred vision, sweating and vomiting. In extreme cases the brain is affected and the person becomes delirious, comatosed and may eventually die.

Dehydration during exercise

Contracting muscles generate a great deal of heat during exercise, up to 100 times more than resting muscles. The body must get rid of this extra heat, or the core body temperature will rise to dangerous levels. The blood transports this heat from the muscles to the skin surface where it is lost through convection, radiation and evaporation (sweating). In hot weather, there is little or no heat loss through convection and radiation, therefore heat loss must be through evaporation with increased sweating.

Vigorous activity produces profuse sweating, which can result in a fluid loss of 4–5 percent of body mass. The longer and harder the exercise and the hotter and more humid the conditions, the greater the fluid loss. Long distance runners may lose as much as two litres every hour through the lungs and skin. As fluid loss increases, the body becomes dehydrated. Water will be lost from all body compartments and there will be a reduction in blood volume. Because there is less blood for the heart to pump per beat, cardiac output is reduced, which in turn reduces the delivery of oxygen and nutrients to the contracting muscles; performance will be limited. The circulatory system tries to maintain blood volume to the muscles by constricting vessels and reducing blood flow to the skin, therefore less heat is lost and temperature rises.

The symptoms of dehydration include: a decrease in level of performance, nausea, irritability, dizziness, fatigue, confusion and eventually complete exhaustion and collapse.

It is possible to prevent dehydration by ensuring an adequate intake of fluid before, during and after vigorous or prolonged activity. Performers are recommended to:

1 Drink plenty of water the day before the event.
2 Drink two cups of water two hours before the event.
3 Drink one cup of water about 15–30 minutes before the event.
4 Drink a quarter to half a cup every 15–20 minutes during the event (this is not necessary for events lasting up to 30 minutes).
5 Rehydrate fully after the event (this will depend on the degree of dehydration).

Recording the weight before and after performance will give an indication of how much water has been lost and how much needs replacing after exercise. For every 1 kilogram of weight lost, 1 litre of water should be drunk to restore balance.

Sports drinks

Drinking water alone may not be enough to rehydrate the body, as the electrolytic balance must also be considered. Drinking water quickly removes the feeling of thirst (to protect against low plasma electrolyte levels), and stimulates the kidneys to excrete urine. This occurs before rehydration is complete. It is important to continue drinking even if feelings of thirst have diminished. Sports drinks are continually being developed, containing sodium and/or carbohydrate (glucose) and other electrolytes. Many of these drinks contain a glucose polymer, which is an easily digestible form of complex carbohydrate. The main aim of these drinks is to speed up rehydration; those containing carbohydrate also maintain blood sugar levels, delay depletion of muscle glycogen, and thus increase endurance.

Research indicates that for athletes exercising at low intensity for up to an hour, water is as effective as expensive sports drinks for preventing dehydration. Exercising for this length of time will not utilise the glucose provided by sports drinks, and the sodium lost is easily replaced through diet.

However, when exercising for long duration at moderate to high intensity, sports drinks are recommended as they rehydrate faster, and if consumed during exercise, can enhance performance. The intake of glucose raises blood sugar levels and spares muscle glycogen, so that the muscles contract harder for longer. Sodium helps to retain water in the blood without inhibiting thirst; it also limits urine production, therefore hydration is faster.

Many nutritionists believe that the diets of most people are already too high in sodium and so do not require it as an addition to drinks. It must also be remembered that carbohydrates supply calories, and those athletes wishing to control weight should avoid the extra calories found in these drinks.

Sports drinks come in different concentrations and selection is important. There are three kinds of sports drinks:

1 hypotonic
2 isotonic
3 hypertonic.

Although all these drinks will rehydrate the body, the main difference lies in their rate of absorption which is dependent on their **osmolarity** (this refers to the concentration of solutes in a solution). A drink with low osmolarity will have fewer particles in solution than a drink with high osmolarity.

Hypotonic drinks

Hypo means: *less* than. These drinks have *low* osmolarity; they have a lower concentration of solutes (less particles), usually less than 4 grams of sugar per 100 ml. They pass quickly out of the stomach and are absorbed for fast rehydration. These are geared to the low/moderate, short duration (up to one hour) athlete. Water would be just as suitable under these conditions, but some will enjoy the flavour of these drinks and consequently drink more.

Isotonic drinks

Iso means: the *same*. These drinks have a higher concentration of solutes than hypotonic drinks and are absorbed at about the same rate as water. They contain 4–8 grams of sugar per 100 ml and will refuel and rehydrate. These drinks are geared to the endurance athlete, exercising for one to three hours; if consumed during performance, they provide extra glycogen.

Hypertonic drinks

Hyper means: *more* than. These drinks have a much higher osmolarity, and are more concentrated than isotonic drinks. They slow gastric emptying, and are absorbed more slowly than water. Containing over 8 grams of sugar per 100 ml, they rehydrate slowly, spare muscle glycogen and prolong endurance. These drinks are geared to the ultramarathon runners, cyclists and others who must maintain effort all day.

Fibre

Fibre provides roughage and bulk which stimulates peristalsis and facilitates the movement of waste through the large intestine for excretion. We obtain fibre from wholemeal foods (brown bread, rice and pasta) and from fruit and vegetables. An intake of 20–35 grams per day is recommended. High fibre intake:

- reduces the risk of heart disease
- helps to lower cholesterol level
- decreases the risk of cancer, particularly colon cancer
- reduces the risk of gastrointestinal problems and diseases
- protects against diabetes.

A high fibre diet must be accompanied by high fluid intake to keep the colon functioning efficiently.

Weight control

Weight control is largely a balance between energy input (food eaten) with energy output (energy used).

- If energy input equals energy output, weight remains stable (neither gained or lost).
- If energy input is greater than energy output, weight increases as the excess fuel is stored on the body as fat.
- If the energy input is less than energy output, weight is lost as fuel is taken from the fat stores.

Therefore the most effective way to lose weight is to eat less and increase the level of aerobic activity. Aerobic exercise is the most effective form of activity for losing weight, as it utilises fat as well as carbohydrate for energy.

Any diet should aim at reducing weight by around 1 kilo per week. It is important to eat a balanced and varied diet and to include each of the foods necessary for health. It is potentially dangerous to reduce calorie intake to 1,000 cals or under. Most people will lose weight on a 1,500–2,000 cals diet. It is worth noting that:

- 1 gram of carbohydrate provides: 4 Kcals (17 kilojoules) of energy.
- 1 gram of protein provides: 4 Kcals (17 kilojoules) of energy.

> but

- 1 gram of fat provides: 9 Kcals (39 kilojoules) of energy.

Therefore, eating more carbohydrate and protein and cutting down on fat will result in less energy intake and quicker weight loss.

Body composition

Body weight is dependent on the major structural components of the body, which include bone, muscle and fat. Weighing machines tell us how heavy we are, and by regularly weighing ourselves, we know whether we have gained or lost weight. We can also compare our weight against the so called 'norm' for our height, by checking established height–weight tables. If our weight is greater than the average values, we are classed as overweight; if our weight is less than the stated values, we are underweight. Being very overweight or very underweight can increase health risks. However, it is important to remember that these are only 'average' values; we may not fit into the 'average mould', and weight alone tells us little about our individual state of health.

The **Body Mass Index (BMI)** is used to assess health risks in relation to weight and height. The BMI is calculated by dividing weight and height. The BMI is calculated by dividing weight in kilograms, by the square of the height in metres. The result is then checked against the following risk table.

Table 9.1 Ranges of body Mass Index					
BMI Males		Diagnosis	BMI Females		
Light frame	Heavy frame		Light frame		Heavy frame
20 – 25		Acceptable	19	–	24
26 – 30		Overweight	25	–	29
31 – 40		Obese	30	–	40
41+		Dangerously obese	41+		

However, body **composition** is the important factor (i.e. the ratio of fat to lean tissue). Too much fat increases the risk of developing many serious diseases such as hypertension, heart disease, vascular problems, stroke, diabetes, gall bladder disease, arthritis and certain cancers.

It is possible to be classed as overweight, even though the percentage of body fat is low. Many athletes and sports people develop large muscles through specific training which will add considerably to their weight. This is desirable weight gain from their point of view, and does not constitute a health problem. They may be overweight when compared with average tables, but they will not be 'overfat', which is the critical issue.

Although diet is the major factor in gaining fat, activity levels play a crucial part, as do other factors such as hormonal influences, inherited characteristics and somatotypes. These factors make it more difficult for some individuals to control their weight:

1 *Endomorphs:* These are short, stocky, curvaceous and plump. For this group weight/fat gain is easy but weight loss is difficult.
2 *Ectomorphs:* These are long limbed, slim and slightly muscular. They do not easily gain weight.
3 *Mesomorphs:* These are muscular and stocky. They gain weight/fat slowly but increase muscle strength easily.

Individuals are predominantly of one type but may have aspects of another.

Summary and aid to learning

Athletes and sportspeople require a low fat to lean tissue ratio, because fat means surplus baggage to carry around. This is costly in terms of energy expenditure which limits endurance. Transporting excess fat will increase inertia, reduce speed and agility. The greater the weight, the greater the inertia and the greater the effort required to overcome it. Fat laid down in muscle tissue increases friction which impairs strength and function. Some athletes and dancers reduce calories to dangerous levels in pursuit of leanness as it is aesthetically desirable and enhances performance.

However, athletes must balance training and diet, and consume extra calories to meet high energy and muscle building requirements, but guard against fat gain.

High carbohydrate, moderate protein, low fat intake is recommended, together with an adequate intake of vitamins, minerals, water and fibre.

Obesity or high fat ratio (i.e., 20 percent over desirable weight) is a major health problem in Western society. The majority of the population is too fat and should change their diet and increase exercise levels. A combination of healthy eating and increased levels of aerobic activity is the key to success. Regular, moderate/low intensity aerobic exercise of 20–30 minutes duration 3–5 times per week combined with reduced calorie intake of around 2,000 calories per day will result in fat loss, improved body shape, and an increase in lean tissue. It is an advantage to have a high proportion of muscle tissue as it has a high metabolic rate, therefore more calories are burnt.

Quick guide to healthy eating

- Reduce intake fat, particularly saturated fat. When cooking boil, steam or bake food; do not fry.
- Reduce intake of red meat as it has high fat content, replace with poultry. Cut off all visible fat from meat and remove the skin from poultry. Avoid eating prepared foods such as sausages, pate, pies, etc.
- Reduce sugar and salt intake.
- Eat plenty of fish, particularly oily fish such as mackerel, salmon, herring, trout.
- Eat plenty of fresh or frozen vegetables – at least five portions per day (but do not overcook).
- Eat plenty of fresh, frozen or dried fruit.
- Eat wholemeal foods such as bread, pasta, rice, cereals, pulses, beans.
- Eat a wide variety of foods.
- Cut down on alcohol.
- Eat plenty of fibre.
- Drink two to three litres of water or diluted fruit juices per day.
- Low fat, high carbohydrate and moderate protein is recommended. Remember that fat has twice the number of calories as carbohydrate and protein (weight for weight).

QUESTIONS

1. Define the following terms
   a basal metabolic rate
   b kilocalorie
   c macronutrients
   d micronutrients
2. List the six basic nutrients necessary for a healthy diet.
3. Explain the importance of including plenty of fibre in the diet.
4. Give six examples of foods which provide carbohydrates.
5. Name the two main types of carbohydrates and give examples of where each is found.
6. Explain why a high carbohydrate intake is vital for distance runners.
7. List the two main types of fat and give examples of where each is found.
8. Compare the energy yield of one gram of fat with one gram of carbohydrate and protein.
9. Explain why a fit person with a high aerobic capacity will burn fat more easily than an unfit person.
10. Explain what is meant by the term 'essential amino acids'.
11. Define the terms:
    a Complete proteins
    b Incomplete proteins.
12. Name the fat soluble vitamins.
13. List four functions of vitamins.
14. Name two important minerals and give their function.
15. Explain what is meant by 'free radicals'. Why are they undesirable in the body?
16. Give three examples of antioxidants and explain their importance in the diet.
17. Explain why water is an important component of the diet.
18. Explain why vigorous exercise may result in dehydration.
19. Give the symptoms of dehydration.
20. Explain the difference between hypotonic, isotonic and hypertonic sports drinks.

Chapter 10
Relaxation and posture

RELAXATION

Relaxation means freedom from tension and anxiety and involves both a physiological and a psychological state. Tension and anxiety are caused by stress, which upsets the body balance, known as homeostasis. The body ceases to function efficiently, resulting in lethargy, illness and disease.

> **LEARN**
> The relaxed state means freedom from tension and anxiety

Stress has been defined as a non-specific response of the body to any demand made on it. Stressors, those factors causing stress, may be social, chemical, bacterial, physical, climatic or psychological. People differ in their ability to cope with stress; some are more affected than others. We are all aware of the symptoms and may well have experienced some ourselves, e.g. increased sweating, increased heart rate, higher blood pressure, rapid breathing, dryness of the mouth, inability to cope, feeling overwhelmed and out of control, inability to concentrate or make decisions, trembling, nail biting, frequent urination, non-stop talking, pacing and other nervous habits.

It is impossible to remove all stressors from daily life. Indeed, a certain degree of stress is desirable and productive, and it can produce feelings of thrill and excitement. However, the ability to relax is very important as it combats stress and reduces its harmful effects. It conserves energy, reduces fatigue, lethargy and overtiredness and helps the body to return to a state of homeostasis.

Allowing the body to rest and recover is essential for those participating in gymnastics, athletics, sport and fitness activities. It is important for all participants in these activities to practise and master relaxation techniques, since the ability to relax at the right moment can improve performance. Total relaxation conserves energy and concentrates the mind before events and so should be practised both before events and during breaks or intervals.

Aids to relaxation

A variety of aids can be used to promote relaxation:

- heat therapy, e.g. heat packs, heat blankets, hot baths, showers, sauna and steam baths and infra-red lamps;
- cold therapy, e.g. cold packs and wraps;
- massage performed in a deep, slow and rhythmic manner;
- preparations such as analgesic liniments, wintergreen and other muscle relaxants.

Relaxation techniques

To achieve long-term benefits, the individual must learn to recognise the difference between being in a tense state and being in a relaxed state. As physical and mental relaxation are interdependent, both must be taught. Although relaxation techniques may appear simple, they are skills that must be learned and practised regularly.

Examples of relaxation techniques:

- The relaxation response
- Progressive relaxation (contract/relax technique)
- Visualisation or imagery
- Biofeedback.

Regardless of the technique, the selection of a warm, quiet environment and the positioning and comfort of the client are important considerations. These factors alone may be sufficient to elicit the relaxation response, as explained below.

Preparation of the room

- The area should be warm and well ventilated.
- The area should be quiet and away from any distracting noises or activities.
- The lighting should be low and diffused.
- The colour scheme should be soft and warming, using pastel colours rather than harsh, bold colours.
- The area should be spotlessly clean and tidy. All linen and towels should be boil-washed and well laundered.

- A comfortable mattress on the floor provides the best support, with pillows for the head and knees. Two low plinths pushed together and covered with a thin mattress can be used. (Clients feel more secure nearer the ground and on a wide rather than a narrow surface.)
- Light blankets can be used for additional warmth.
- Very soft relaxing music may be played in the background. This depends on client preference, as some clients do not like absolute quiet and become tense.

Client care

A full client consultation should be carried out.

- Allow the client time to discuss their lifestyle and any problems that may be contributing to stress and anxiety levels.
- Discuss stress levels at work or during sport or training that may be affecting performance. Advise and suggest strategies for coping where possible. Explain how relaxation will help.
- Suggest suitable clothing, such as a loose-fitting cotton vest, T-shirt or sweater and loose-fitting pyjama or track suit bottoms. Loose socks can be worn on the feet. (Do not allow the client to walk around in socks as there is a danger of slipping.)
- If suitable clothing is not available, loosen the clothing, remove the tie and belt, loosen the collar and trousers or skirt and remove the shoes.
- Suggest that the client uses the toilet, as it is impossible to relax with a full bladder.
- Use some form of heat, if available, prior to the commencement of relaxation training. (Follow the correct procedure when applying heat.)
- Create an atmosphere conducive to relaxation. Smile, be calm, pleasant and relaxed, speak slowly and clearly, keep your voice low and do not rush or hurry the client. Explain the procedure clearly and carefully to alleviate any anxiety.

> ### LEARN
> Create an atmosphere conducive to relaxation. Allow the client time to talk and explain their problems. Listen attentively and quietly.

The relaxation response

The client relaxes in response to four basic conditions:

- a quiet environment – this cuts out noise, limits distraction and allows the individual to switch off;
- a comfortable position – the position selected for all relaxation techniques is very important. The position should be selected to suit the preference of the client: lying, half lying or the recovery position may be chosen. The body must be well supported with pillows to minimise muscle effort and to enable the client to remain in this position for a considerable length of time;
- mental concentration – this can be an image on which to concentrate, such as a sphere, box or vase, or any object in the room, such as a clock or mirror. The client concentrates hard on this one image and empties the mind of other thoughts or images;

■ a passive attitude – this is the most difficult, especially for those with extreme mental anxiety. It involves letting go and emptying the mind of thoughts and distractions.

Progressive relaxation

This method was developed by Dr. Edmund Jacobson, one of the pioneers in the field of relaxation. It aims to develop an awareness of the difference between feelings of tension and relaxation within muscles and muscle groups. The client is taught to contract and relax each muscle group in sequence, from the foot to the head. With practice, the client will appreciate the difference between being tense and relaxed and will develop the ability to adopt the relaxed state quickly. The client can then be taught to recognise differing degrees of tension within muscles by using the same sequence but varying the contraction, from full contraction to part contraction and minimal contraction, for each muscle or group.

The therapist should select a suitable venue and prepare the client (see page 00). The client should lie on a mattress and be fully supported. Modifications of the lying position can be used, for example the recovery position, with the body well supported with pillows, the supine position (on the back) with a pillow under the head and knees, or half lying, with pillows for the head and knees. Encourage the client to 'let go', breathe deeply and close the eyes gently.

The technique is then practised as follows, beginning with the feet and repeating each movement three times:
■ Pull the feet up hard (dorsi-flexion), then let go.
■ Push the feet down hard (plantar flexion), then let go.
■ Push the knees down hard against the floor, then let go.
■ Push the leg down hard against the floor, then let go.
■ Tighten the buttock muscles hard, then let go.
■ Pull the abdominal muscles in hard, then let go.
■ Raise the shoulders off the floor, then let go.
■ Press the shoulders hard into the floor, then let go.
■ Press the arms hard into the floor, then let go.
■ Curl the fingers to make a fist, then let go.
■ Press the head into the floor, then let go.
■ Screw up and tighten the face, then let go.
■ Tighten all groups, then let go.

The client should breathe out as he or she 'lets go'.

The therapist must use her voice to good effect when teaching relaxation. The command 'tighten hard' should be firm, and 'let go' should be spoken in a lower tone and drawn out longer to encourage the feeling of letting go. The terms 'relax' and 'release' can be used or interchanged with 'let go'.

Clients can then practise the sequence on their own until they are free of tension and sleepy. They should be left for 15 to 20 minutes and then woken up slowly.

As clients develop the ability they can be taught to appreciate differing degrees of tension. This is done in the same way as above, except that the first contraction should be maximal, the second contraction partial and the third contraction minimal. The commands would be as follows:

- Pull the feet up hard, and relax.
- Gently pull the feet up, just feel the muscle pulling, and relax.
- Move the foot upwards ever so slightly, and relax.

Clients should then practise the three different contractions in their own time, feeling the difference in muscle tension each time.

The therapist will work through the body in this way, using the same sequence as above.

TASK
Work with a partner.
- Position your partner comfortably in the recovery position, using pillows as required.
- Teach your partner to relax using the progressive relaxation technique.

Visualisation or imagery

This technique requires the individual to visualise situations or conditions conducive to relaxation. For example:

- Imagine lying on the beach in warm sunshine. It is quiet and peaceful, you feel warm and heavy.
- Imagine lying in a field in warm sunshine. You smell the grass. You feel warm and heavy.
- Imagine sinking into a feather duvet. It feels soft and warm and wraps around you.
- Think of any situation that recalls warmth, comfort and peace.
- Concentrate entirely on the rhythm of breathing, letting the breathing become deeper and slower.

Any examples that enhance relaxation can be included.

Visualisation with breathing can be used to good effect when performing static-stretch and flexibility exercises that require the relaxed state.

The client should exhale and move into the stretch position, stretching until tension is felt in the muscle belly. This position is held while the client breathes in and out slowly for a few cycles. The client then breathes in then out slowly while moving into a further stretch, imagining the muscle fibres letting go and lengthening. When tension develops the position is held briefly, followed by relaxation.

Biofeedback

When it is difficult to appreciate the difference between muscle tension and relaxation, biofeedback techniques using special equipment may be applied. The equipment gives a reading that relates to the degree of tension, and the mind is then used to attempt a change in the reading.

POSTURE

Posture is the term used to describe the alignment of the body, in other words how the body is held. Good posture means that the body is balanced and the muscle work required to maintain an upright position is minimal. Poor posture means that the body is out of balance and certain muscles must contract strongly to maintain this position. Over time, this means that those muscles will tighten and shorten, while others weaken and stretch. This muscle imbalance imposes stresses on the underlying structures, the ligaments and joints, resulting in deformities, stiffness and pain. The body loses its ability to function at maximum efficiency and the performance of everyday activities, movement and exercise can become severely limited.

Poor alignment of one part of the body can affect other parts. This can be more clearly understood if we think of the body in terms of segments. Each segment must be perfectly balanced on the one below. If one segment moves forwards, backwards or sideways, adjustments have to be made in all the other segments for balance to be restored.

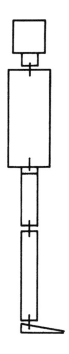

FIGURE NUMBER: 10.1 – Body segments must be balanced one on the other.

Posture is dynamic, constantly adjusting to counteract the forces acting upon the body. Postural adjustments may be made consciously or unconsciously. The cerebral cortex, basal nuclei, cerebellum and brain stem all play a part in the control of posture.

These higher centres respond to different impulses arriving from various sensory receptors. Information on the body's position in space is received from muscle spindles, from tendon and joint receptors, from the eyes and ears and from the skin on the soles of the feet. The higher centres respond to incoming information and relay impulses back to the muscles, initiating muscle contraction to produce corrective action.

Posture is influenced by many factors, both physical and psychological. A large proportion of the population leads a sedentary life and takes little exercise, which leads to muscle imbalance and poor body alignment. Other factors that influence posture include heredity, weight distribution, height, nervous tension, illness, fatigue, occupational stress, poor working conditions and poor sitting positions. Psychological and emotional states also have an effect – people who are happy, confident and extrovert, with high self-esteem, exhibit good posture, while those who are unhappy, sad, introverted and lacking in confidence, with low self-esteem, have poor posture.

Poor posture results in muscle imbalance. Some muscles become tight, while others will be overstretched. This imposes stress on the ligaments, tendons and underlying joints, producing pain and stiffness. In addition, certain muscles are unable to work through their full range. This not only restricts the activities of daily living but severely limits the capacity to perform at maximum potential in athletics, sports, dancing, etc.

Poor posture affects general health. The natural movements of the thorax may be restricted and its expansion limited, which results in shallow breathing. This reduces the intake of oxygen and the elimination of carbon dioxide. The circulation is affected due to the tension in muscles and the reduction in thoracic movement, which mean that blood is unable to flow freely around the body. This limits the delivery of nutrients and the elimination of waste products.

Good postural habits should be developed when young and maintained throughout life. It is possible to improve posture for all age groups through appropriate exercise. The extent of the improvement will depend on the degree of deformity, the age and the commitment of the individual.

Good posture is important for the following reasons:
- maintaining muscle balance;
- improving body shape and appearance;
- preventing muscle tension, spasm and pain;
- preventing stresses on ligaments, tendons and joints;
- preventing skeletal deformities and associated pain;
- increasing the movement of the thorax, resulting in deeper breathing with an increase in oxygen intake and the elimination of carbon dioxide;
- improving the efficiency of the circulatory system;

- improving the performance of all activities and exercises and enhancing peak performance;
- reducing the risk of musculo-skeletal injuries.

Evaluation of posture

Posture must be accurately examined and evaluated before correction can take place. An accurate assessment of posture should form part of the client consultation. All findings should be carefully recorded and appropriate exercises devised for correction of the faults.

Aids to postural assessment

The following aids can be used to make assessment easier and more accurate.

- a plumb line to check body alignment;
- a mirror to provide visual feedback for the client. First, look at the client's normal posture and discuss any problem areas. Correct the posture and discuss the improvements. View the posture from the front, side and back. On the front view, lines can be drawn to check the level of the ear lobes and shoulders, the waist angles, and the level of the right and left anterior superior iliac spines and the knees. On the side view, draw a vertical line from the ear lobe to just in front of the lateral malleolus – does it fall through the plumb-line points? Check for round shoulders, kyphosis, lordosis, flat back, sway back and hyper-extended knees. On the back view, check for winged scapulae, scoliosis, pelvic level and buttock folds.
- a graphed board – the client stands in front of the board and the relevant bony points (ear lobes, shoulders, waist angles, knees) are marked, examined for any deviation and discussed.

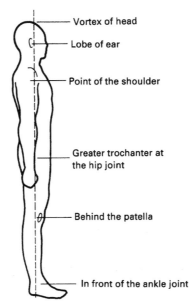

Vortex of head

Lobe of ear

Point of the shoulder

Greater trochanter at the hip joint

Behind the patella

In front of the ankle joint

FIGURE NUMBER: 10.2 – Points that the line of gravity will pass through when posture is correct.

It is not necessary to use all these aids, but one or two will help the client to appreciate his or her problems.

Procedure

- Welcome and observe the client as she/he walks into the room.
- Ask the client to sit, observing how he or she sits down.
- Take the client's details – names, address, doctor's address, medical history, occupation. Discuss fully any stresses at work, working positions, seating, etc. Discuss lifestyle, associated activities, and nutritional standards. Try to assess the client's psychological state while talking – is he or she tense, under stress, fatigued or exhausted? Is the client an introvert or extrovert, or are there any other factors that might influence posture?
- Ask the client to undress down to pants only, making sure that there is complete privacy.
- If possible observe the posture as the client walks around the room (this may not be possible in a small cubicle). Many problems can be observed when the body is in motion. Observe the client sitting down and standing up: are the movements evenly balanced or does he or she sit and stand unevenly?
- Ask the client to adopt a normal stance and assess the posture from the front, side and back.
- Discuss any problem areas with the client. Stand him or her in front of a mirror, indicate the postural faults and show how they may be corrected.
- Correct the client's posture and ask him or her to hold the adjustments until good posture is obtained (the new positioning will seem very unnatural at first).
- Tell the client to relax and then to make the adjustments independently and hold the corrected stance.
- Explain to the client that frequent practice is needed throughout the day.
- Teach appropriate exercises to restore muscle balance.

The examination of posture

From the front
Head position:
- Are the ear lobes level? If they are not there is muscle imbalance. The sterno-cleido-mastoid and the upper fibres of the trapezius are tight on the lower side, while those on the other side will be stretched.

Shoulders:
- Are they level, or is one higher than the other, indicating muscle imbalance? The upper fibres of the trapezius and levator scapulae are tight on the raised side. A difference in level may also indicate scoliosis, so check for that also. (A slight difference is considered normal.)
- Are both shoulders held high? This indicates tension in the muscles on both sides. The right and left upper fibres of the trapezius and the levator scapulae are tight.

- Are the shoulders drawn forwards, rounded? This indicates muscle imbalance. The pectoral muscles are tight but the middle fibres of the trapezius and the rhomboids are stretched.
- Are there hollows above the clavicles? This indicates muscle tension, which may be due to respiratory problems such as asthma.

Breasts:
- Are the breasts held high or sagging? If there is breast sag and round shoulders, correction of the posture may help to lift the breasts.

Waist:
- Are the waist angles on the right and left level? If one is lower than the other, there may be spinal deformity or a difference in leg length.

Anterior superior iliac spines:
- Are they level? If not, there may be spinal deformity or a difference in leg length.
- Are they dropped forward? This indicates a lordosis with a tight erector spinae and quadratus lumborum and weak abdominals.
- Are they dropped backwards? This indicates a flat back or sway back, with weak back extensors, i.e. the erector spinae and quadratus lumborum, and tight abdominals.

Patellae:
- Do they point forwards? If not there may be knock knees (genu valgum) or bow legs (genu varum).

Toes:
- Do they point forwards? If they point outwards there may be flattening of the medial arch and flat feet.
- If they point inwards or outwards, the weight distribution over the foot will be wrong, causing foot problems.
- Look for bunions, where the big toe deviates towards and sometimes across the other toes and there is swelling at the metatarso-phalangeal joint.
- Look for hammer toes, where the inter-phalangeal joints are deformed.

From the side

Use a plumb line. This should fall through the lobe of the ear, the point of the shoulder and the hip joint, behind the patella and just in front of the lateral malleolus.

Head position:
- Is the neck or cervical curve exaggerated and the chin forward? This means that the neck extensors, the upper fibres of the trapezius at the back of the neck, are tight and the neck flexors are weak.

Thoracic curve:
- Is there kyphosis, i.e. an exaggerated thoracic curve, giving a humped look? This means that the pectoral muscles are tight and the middle fibres of the trapezius and rhomboids are weak.

Abdomen:
- Is the abdomen protruding or sagging forwards, indicating weakness of the abdominal muscles? The pelvis may be tilted forward. This is known as visceroptosis as the weak abdominals allow the viscera to sag forward.

Lumbar curve:

■ Is there lordosis, i.e. an exaggerated lumbar curve with the spine curved inwards? This means that there will be an anterior pelvic tilt with weak abdominals and a tight erector spinae and quadratus lumborum.

■ If the lumbar region is flat, which is much less common, the erector spinae and quadratus lumborum will be weak.

Buttocks:

■ Are the buttocks well toned with strong muscles, or are the gluteal muscles weak and sagging?

Knees:

■ Are the knees hyper-extended?

From the back

Head:

■ Are the ear lobes level or is the head tilted, indicating muscle imbalance? (See front.)

Shoulders:

■ Are they level? (See front.)

■ Are there winged scapulae, i.e. the inferior angle and medial border of the scapulae lift away from the chest wall? This indicates a weakness of the serratus anterior and the lower fibres of the trapezius.

Spine:

■ Is there scoliosis, i.e. a lateral deviation of the spine? This may be an S or C curve to the right or left. If you are unsure, pull a finger firmly down the spinous processes: the red line should be straight, and will show up any deviation. A scoliosis may be structural (present from birth). Or it may be postural, and will straighten out when the body is flexed forward.

Buttocks:

■ Are the buttock folds level? If they are not, scoliosis, lateral pelvic tilt or different leg length may be present.

Heels:

■ Are these square and firmly planted on the ground? If not, the weight distribution will be uneven.

Correction of the posture

The correction of the posture should begin at the feet. Each position should be maintained as the subsequent one is practised.

Feet

Stand with the feet four to six inches apart, with the toes pointing forward. The weight should be evenly distributed between the balls of the feet and the heels.

Practise the following:

■ Raise the toes off the ground, feel the weight evenly distributed between the balls and heels, then lower the toes.

- Sway the body forwards, feeling more weight on the balls.
- Sway the body backwards, feeling more weight on the heels.
- Position the body so that the weight is evenly distributed between the balls and the heels. Lift the medial arch slightly, but do not curl the toes.

Knees

- Press the knees backwards hard, ease the knees by bending them slightly, then find the mid-point and pull the kneecaps upwards by tightening the quadriceps muscle.
- If the knees are hyper-extended, ease them slightly and pull the kneecaps upwards as above.
- If the knees are bowed or knock-kneed, tighten the kneecaps, rotate the thighs outwards and tighten the buttocks to bring the kneecaps to point forward.

Check the feet again after performing these movements.

Pelvis

Tilt the pelvis forwards and then backwards; pull it forwards again slightly, tucking the tail under, and hold this balance. Pull the abdomen in and breathe out as the pelvis is pulled forward, then hold this position while breathing normally.

Thorax

Pull the thorax upwards from the waist as you breathe in, drawing the shoulders backwards and downwards. Hold this position while breathing normally. Do not thrust the chest forwards.

Neck and head

Elongate the neck and pull the chin backwards. Feel as though someone is pulling the hair upwards at the crown.

Check the feet, knees, pelvis and thorax again, hold this position and then relax.

Practise this correction several times a day and during various activities; correct the posture during inhalation and hold the balance during exhalation.

If the new posture is maintained while walking around, it will eventually become habitual.

Summary and aid to learning

Relaxation means being free from tension and anxiety which are normally caused by stress.

Aids to relaxation include any form of mild heat, cold packs, slow deep massage, analgesic ointments and types of muscle relaxants.

List the sources of heat that could be used to promote relaxation.

The preparation of the room is very important.

Prepare a room or cubicle for a client needing to practise relaxation.

Relaxation techniques include:

The relaxation response involves the client's response to a quiet soothing environment, total concentration on a particular object while trying to let go of all tension.

Progressive relaxation aims to develop an awareness of the difference between feelings of tension and relaxation. Contraction, relaxation of all the large muscle groups is performed working systematically around the body.

Visualisation or imagery involves visualising situations or conditions conducive to relaxation.

Biofeedback involves a meter which registers tension; the client then attempts through will power to lower the tension.

Practise these relaxation techniques with a partner.

Posture refers to the alignment of the body.

The upright posture is maintained by the contraction of the postural muscles.

List the postural muscles.

Poor alignment of one part will impose stresses on other parts.

Poor posture may affect health, as the movement of the thorax may be restricted; this will reduce oxygen intake. The tension of the shortened muscles and restricted movement of the thorax will adversly affect the blood flow around the body.

Give reasons why good posture is important.

Postural problems include:
Kyphosis: an exaggerated thoracic curve.
Lordosis: an exaggerated lumbar curve. Lordosis may be accompanied by the condition known as visceroptosis which occurs when the abdominal muscles are very weak and the viscera protrude forward.
Kypho–lordosis is a combination of the above, where both thoracic and lumbar curves are exaggerated.
Scoliosis is a long C-shaped or an S-shaped lateral deviation of the vertebral column.
Flat back refers to a loss of the lumbar curve resulting in a flat back.

QUESTIONS

1. List some aids which may be used to promote relaxation.
2. Explain why rest is important between training sessions.
3. Explain the factors which must be considered when preparing the room for relaxation.
4. List four basic conditions which promote the relaxation response.
5. Describe the positioning of the client prior to teaching relaxation.
6. Describe briefly how you would teach progressive relaxation technique.
7. Explain how breathing and visualisation may be used to promote relaxation.
8. Briefly explain the effect of inadequate rest and relaxation on the sportsperson.
9. Give six effects of poor posture.
10. Describe the use of any two 'aids' which may be used when assessing posture.
11. List all the points that a plumb line must pass through, if posture is correct.
12. Describe the postural problem 'kyphosis', and indicate which muscles are involved.
13. Name the condition associated with anterior pelvic tilt.
14. Give six exercises for the correction of each of the following conditions:
    a round shoulders
    b lordosis
    c flat back.
15. Name the weak muscles associated with 'winged scapula'. Give four exercises to strengthen these muscles.

TASKS

Work with a partner. Carry out a role with one of you as the client and one as the therapist.
- Greet the client and carry out a consultation.
- Assess the posture using the plumb line.
- Teach the correction of the posture.

Chapter 11
Specific exercise for correction of postural problems

Specific exercise programmes may be required to mobilise joints, to strengthen specific muscles or to correct postural faults.

The objectives must be clearly stated and explained to the client. Once she is familiar with the exercises the client should be encouraged to practise them at home. Careful analysis of the problem areas is necessary so that the appropriate corrective strategy may be worked out. The following are possible exercises for the correction of common problems.

Consider the starting positions carefully. Younger clients can use standing or modifications of standing, but older clients will be more stable if sitting or lying. Older clients, or those with painful or arthritic knee joints, should not be placed in the kneeling position.

> **LEARN**
> Consider the starting position, carefully select the stability to suit the client. Avoid stressing painful joints

In addition, read the sections on strengthening and stretching, the warm-up and the cooldown in chapter 9. Any appropriate exercises may be selected from those listed, or you may add some of your own. Remember that strength will only improve if the muscle is made to work progressively harder. The intensity of the exercises should increase gradually to peak intensity and decrease gradually. This applies to the warm-up and the main scheme.

THE POSTURAL CORRECTION OF LORDOSIS

This is an exaggerated curve of the lumbar spine where the pelvis is tilted forward.

The weak muscles that require strengthening are:
the abdominals – these are the rectus abdominus, the internal oblique and the external oblique – and the hip extensors – the hamstrings and the gluteus maximus.

The tight muscles that require stretching are
the trunk extensors – the erector spinae and quadratus lumborum – and
the hip flexors, particularly the ilio-psoas.

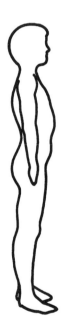

FIGURE NUMBER: 11.1 – Lordosis.

Aims of the treatment

- To strengthen the abdominals, thus pulling the pelvis upwards and backwards
- To strengthen the hip extensors
- To stretch the erector spinae and quadratus lumborum
- To stretch the hip flexors.

Remember to use crook lying as a starting position for the abdominal strengthening and to keep the small of the back against the floor.

Exercises for the correction of lordosis

Read the appropriate suggestions for strengthening and stretching.

Warm-up – include exercises for mobilising, pulse raising and short stretch

Starting position	Exercise
■ Crook lying	tilt pelvis upwards pressing lumbar region into the floor, release.
■ Crook lying	keeping the chin in, raise the head and shoulders to look at the knees.
■ Crook lying	curl up. This is progressed by moving the hand position to head rest and then stretching above the head.
■ Bend crook lying	twist the trunk, bringing alternate elbows to the opposite knee.
■ Yard crook lying	drop the knees to the right and then to the left.
■ Lying	slide the right arm down the right side and the left arm down the left side.
■ Prone kneeling	arch the back to stretch the lumbar spine, then return to horizontal.
■ Prone kneeling	stretch alternate legs out and lift no more than fifteen degrees above horizontal.

THE POSTURAL CORRECTION OF KYPHOSIS

This is an exaggerated curve of the thoracic region. The shoulders are usually rounded, the neck is shortened and held in extension and the chin pokes forward.

The weak muscles that require strengthening are:
the middle fibres of the trapezius, the rhomboids and the erector spinae.

The tight muscles that require stretching are:
the pectoralis major and the neck extensors.

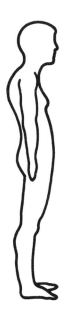

FIGURE NUMBER: 11.2 – Kyphosis.

Aims of the treatment

■ To strengthen the shoulder retractors, namely the middle fibres of the trapezius and the rhomboids, thus drawing the shoulders backwards
■ To strengthen the erector spinae to maintain the erect posture
■ To stretch the pectoralis major.

Remember that many of these exercises are also used to correct round shoulders.

Always keep the chin in and maintain a long neck when performing these exercises.

Exercises for the correction of kyphosis

Warm-up – mobilisers, pulse raisers, stretch

Starting position	Exercise
■ Standing	hold posture correction.
■ Stride standing	gently drop the head forward, pulling the chin in. Press the head back, making a long neck, and raise.

■ Lax stoop sitting	raise the trunk gradually from the base of the spine, vertebra by vertebra.
■ Lax stoop sitting	as above, against resistance from the therapist.
■ Stride standing	circle the shoulders backwards.
■ Stride standing	circle the arms backwards.
■ Stride standing	pull the shoulders backwards.
■ Across bend stride standing	pull the shoulders back and release. Then pull the elbows back and release. Then press the arms back and release.
■ Lax stoop stride standing	slowly return to standing from the base of the spine, vertebra by vertebra.
■ Stoop standing	clasp the hands behind the back, pull the arms and shoulders up and back, hold for a count of ten and release.
■ Crook lying	place a tightly rolled towel lengthways along the spine between the scapulae, press the shoulders back towards the floor, hold for a count of ten and release.
■ Crook lying, arms out to side, elbows at right angles, palms facing forward	as above.
■ Prone lying	keeping the chin in, pull the shoulders back and raise the head and shoulders
■ Prone lying, hands clasped behind the back	pull on the hands and pull the shoulders off the floor.
■ Prone lying, hands clasped behind back	keeping the chin in, pull the shoulders back, lifting the head and shoulders off the floor.
■ Wing prone lying	keeping the chin in, lift the head and shoulders off the floor, pulling the shoulders back.

■ Wing prone lying

as above, but against the resistance of the therapist.

■ Prone lying

with the arms abducted, elbows bent and palms to the floor, lift the arms and head and shoulders.

■ Yard prone lying

as above.

■ Sitting

place one hand behind the neck and the other behind the back, and try to clasp hands or link with a strap. Pull downwards, bringing the upper arm nearer the head, hold for a count of ten and release.

■ Sitting

use a bar that is shoulder-width long. Hold the bar at the ends, lift it upwards above the head and then lower it down behind the head. Hold for a count of ten and lift up.

Kypho-lordosis is a combination of the previous two conditions. Select exercises from the two schemes for this condition.

THE POSTURAL CORRECTION OF ROUND SHOULDERS

In this condition the shoulders are protracted (drawn forward), the head is extended and the chin pokes forward.

This postural defect may be present without any kyphosis of the spine. However, if the spine is kyphotic the shoulders will also be rounded.

The weak muscles that require strengthening are:
the middle fibres of the trapezius and the rhomboids.

The tight muscles that require stretching are:
the pectorals and the neck extensors.

Aims of the treatment

- To strengthen the shoulder retractors and draw the shoulders backwards
- To stretch the pectoralis major and the neck extensors.

For suitable exercises, refer to the scheme for kyphosis. The same exercises can be used for both conditions.

You may wish to modify this slightly by selecting others from chapters 9 and this chapter or by adding your own.

THE POSTURAL CORRECTION OF SCOLIOSIS

This is a lateral curvature of the spine, which may be a long C curve or an S curve. The condition may cause scapular deviation and slight unevenness in the levels of the shoulders and pelvic girdle, caused by muscle imbalance on the right and left sides of the spine. The spine must be carefully examined. To make observation easier, run a finger downwards along the spinous processes with slight pressure. The red line will show the extent and direction of the curve. If the condition is postural, the curve will right itself in forward flexion; ask the client to bend over so that you can see if this is so. If the condition does not correct with flexion it is a structural problem and should be referred to a doctor.

The muscles that will require strengthening will be those on the outside of the curve.

The muscles that will require stretching will be those on the inside of the curve.

General back-strengthening exercises are usually effective in correcting this condition. It is frequently found in adolescence, when pupils carry heavy school bags over the same shoulder or in the same hand each day. Suggest that the bag is carried in one hand to school and in the other on the way home.

Aims of the treatment

To restore balance to muscles of the back, thus reducing the deformity.

Exercises for the correction of Scoliosis

Warm-up – mobilising, pulse raising and stretch

Starting position	Exercise
■ Stride standing	reach up into the air with the hand on the concave side of the curve, where the muscles are tight, and reach towards the floor with the other hand. Stretch, hold, relax, repeat.
■ Stride standing	side flex the trunk towards the convex side, where the muscles are stretched. Slide the hand down the side and return.
■ Prone lying	stretch the arm up along the floor on the concave side and slide the arm down the side of convexity. Hold, release and repeat.
■ Prone lying	stretch the arm above the head on the concave side and the opposite leg along the floor.
■ Prone lying	raise the opposite arm and leg as above.
■ Crook lying, arms abducted and elbows at right angles, palms to floor	rotate the arms to palms up and push back into the floor.
■ Prone lying, arms abducted and elbows at right angles, palms to floor	raise arms backwards.
■ Prone lying, arms to side	keeping the chin in, lift the head and shoulders.
■ Prone lying, clasping hands behind back	keeping the chin in, lift the head and shoulders and pull down the arms.
■ Prone lying, arms abducted, elbows at right angles, palms to floor	raise the arms, head and shoulders. (Do not extend the head; keep it in line with the body.)
■ Yard prone lying	as above.
■ Stretch prone lying	as above.

THE POSTURAL CORRECTION OF FLAT BACK

This is a condition where there is little or no lumbar curve, the back is flat in this region and the pelvis is tilted backwards. It is usually accompanied by kyphosis of the thoracic spine.

The muscles that require strengthening are:
the back extensors, namely the erector spinae. (Sometimes the abdominals and gluteus maximus are weak.)

The muscles that require stretching are:
the hamstrings.

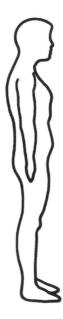

FIGURE NUMBER: 11.3 – Flat back.

Aims of the treatment

- To try to develop a normal lumbar curve by strengthening the erector spinae and gluteus maximus
- To maintain a correct pelvic tilt by ensuring the strength of the abdominals and stretch of the hamstrings.

Exercises for the correction of flat back

Warm-up – mobilisers, pulse raisers and stretch

Starting position	Exercise
■ Sitting	lean forward, taking the pressure from the buttocks onto the thigh, then extend the back to create a lumbar lordosis. Hold for a count of ten and release.
■ Prone lying	raise alternate legs.
■ Prone lying	raise both legs (allowed for this condition).
■ Prone kneeling	arch and hollow the back.
■ Prone kneeling	lift alternate legs up and backwards, stretch, hold and return to the floor.
■ Lying with rolled towel under lumbar spine	flex one knee, then extend the leg up towards the ceiling. Keep the opposite leg pressed hard down on the floor. Repeat with the other leg.
■ Long sitting	rotate the pelvis forwards, then lean slightly backwards. Hold and release.
■ Supine lying, legs up against a wall, with a towel under lumbar spine	pull alternate legs away from the wall, keeping the knee straight and the pelvis on the floor. Hold and release.

THE CORRECTION OF FLABBY UPPER ARMS

This is due to poor muscle tone in the triceps, which is the extensor muscle of the elbow. Fatty deposits in this area also contribute to the problem.

The muscle that requires strengthening is the triceps. If the client is overweight, he or she will need aerobic work to reduce the percentage of body fat.

Aims of the treatment

■ To increase the strength of the triceps muscle
■ To reduce body fat if necessary.

Remember that the triceps extends the elbow joint; therefore, elbow extension must be the movement that is included in all exercises for improving this condition. Movement downwards is assisted by gravitational pull and uses the biceps, working eccentrically, to control the movement, therefore triceps is not working. Movements using the triceps must therefore be horizontal or upwards.

Exercises for the correction of flabby upper arms

Warm-up – mobilisers, pulse raisers and stretch
If the client needs to lose weight, include an aerobic section here for 20 minutes.

Starting position	Exercise
■ Across bend sitting or stride standing	stretch alternate arms out sideways and back; stretch both arms out sideways and back.
■ Bend stride standing	punch forward; punch a pillow or punch bag.
■ Stride standing	place the hands against the therapist's hands, with elbows bent. Push alternate arms straight against the therapist's resistance.
■ Bend stride standing or sitting	stretch the arm vertically upwards. Repeat with progressive weights.
■ Stride standing, arms bent, hands against a wall, leaning forwards	push away from the wall.
■ Prone kneeling	bend and straighten the elbows.
■ Prone lying	place the hands under the shoulders and push up.
■ Prone lying	press-ups.
■ Lean sitting holding weights	holding the weight in the hand at shoulder level, extend the arm backwards and upwards.

■ Crook lying

holding the weight in the hands at shoulder level, push the weights vertically upward and then lower. The weights can be increased for progression.

THE CORRECTION OF WINGED SCAPULA

This is a condition where the medial border and inferior angle of the scapula move back away from the chest wall. It is due to weakness of the serratus anterior and the lower fibres of the trapezius.

Muscles that require strengthening are:
the serratus anterior and the lower fibres of the trapezius.

Aims of the treatment

■ To strengthen those muscles which hold the scapula against the chest wall.

Remember that the serratus anterior is used powerfully in all punching movements. It helps the trapezius to swing the scapula laterally during arm abduction and arm swinging, and it works powerfully to hold the scapula in position when the weight of the body is taken on the hands, as in prone kneeling, push-ups and press-ups.

The exercises for strengthening this muscle are the same as those for strengthening the triceps.

THE CORRECTION OF FLABBY BUTTOCKS

These are caused by poor muscle tone in the hip extensors, primarily the gluteus maximus. The hip abductors also contribute to the problem, namely the gluteus medius, gluteus minimus and tensor fascia lata.

The muscles that require strengthening are:
the hip extensors, i.e. the gluteus maximus, the hamstrings, and the hip abductors.

The muscles that require stretching are:
the hip flexors, primarily the ilio-psoas.

Aims of the treatment

■ To increase the strength of the hip extensors and abductors
■ To stretch the hip flexors.

Remember that the hip extensors will extend the fully flexed hip backwards until the leg is in line with the body and for a further fifteen degrees. At this point further movement is prevented by the structure and ligaments of the hip joint and by the tension in the flexors. The hip extensors will also pull the forward-flexed trunk upwards, working with origin and insertion reversed.

Exercises for the correction of flabby buttocks

Warm-up – mobilisers, pulse raisers, stretch

Starting position	Exercise
■ High sitting	tighten the buttocks.
■ High sitting	press the thighs downwards into the seat and rotate them outwards.
■ Forward stoop sitting	raise the trunk upwards against the resistance of the therapist.
■ Stoop stride standing, hands on legs	raise the trunk to standing.
■ Crook lying	tighten the buttocks and raise the pelvis.
■ Prone kneeling	stretch alternate legs out behind. Attach ankle weights for progression. (Caution: do not arch the back or lift the leg more than fifteen degrees above horizontal.)
■ Side lying	swing the upper leg forward and back.
■ Side lying	push back against resistance from the therapist or springs.
■ Side lying	raise and lower the upper leg, using weights for progression.
■ Prone lying	bending the knee, raise alternate legs off the floor.
■ Prone lying	raise alternate straight legs off the floor (Caution: extend the leg fifteen degrees only and keep the hips on the floor.) Use weights for progression.
■ Prone lying on a couch with one leg over the edge	lift leg backwards and upwards fifteen degrees from horizontal. Use weights for progression. Repeat with the other leg.

TASKS

Work with a partner. Practise a role play with one of you as the client and the other as the therapist.

- ■ Select one of the postural problems – the 'client' mimics this standing posture.
- ■ Identify the weak muscles for strengthening and the tight muscles for stretching.
- ■ Construct a scheme of exercises to correct the problem.
- ■ Teach the exercises to the client.

PART C

Safety Considerations, Assessment and exercise guidelines

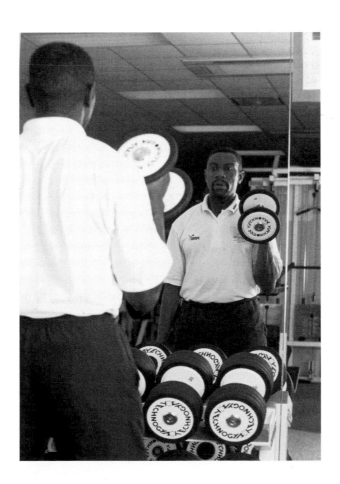

Chapter 12
General exercises

WARM-UP

Performing a warm-up routine prior to any active performance is an important safety factor. The warm-up is designed to prepare the body systems for more intense activity. It allows the systems to make gradual adaptations in preparation for increased demand. This is very important for the cardiovascular system as it cannot adapt quickly and a change from a sedentary, relaxed state to high level activity will impose a stress on the heart. A warm-up should last for 15–20 minutes but environmental temperature should be considered. On cold days a longer warm-up routine will be required. It should be long enough to produce a warm feeling and induce light sweating. This is a good indication that the body temperature has been raised sufficiently to begin the stretch routine. The intensity of the movements should increase gradually and decrease gradually. To bring about the desired adaptations the warm-up should include:

pulse raisers are any aerobic activity which will raise the heart rate gradually. They must begin with low level, slow activity which gradually increases in intensity.

mobilising exercises which improve the range of movement at the joints. Initially the joints are moved through middle range. As the warm-up continues the range is gradually increased through to full range.

stretch/flexibility are performed to improve the extensibility and elasticity of muscles, ligaments and tendons. This may limit or prevent injury as these tissues are more able to accommodate any excessive forces imposed upon them.

After these activities, athletes and sports people include specific movements or routines relevant to the performances e.g. tennis players practise the serve etc.

Warm-up is performed for both physiological and psychological effects.

Physiological effects of warm-up

- Increase in heart rate and dilation of capillaries which will increase blood flow to the active muscles.
- Increased blood flow to active muscles through blood shunting (the volume of blood to the viscera is reduced and redirected to active muscles). This will increase the delivery of glycogen and oxygen to the muscles and removal of metabolic waste from the muscles.
- Increased body and muscle temperature.
- Increased enzyme activity and increased metabolic rate due to temperature rise will ensure a continuing supply of energy.
- Increased elasticity and extensibility of warm muscles will improve speed and force of contraction.
- Increased extensibility of connective tissue components, ligaments and tendons will reduce the risk of injury.
- Increased speed of nerve impulse transmission which will improve skill componants.
- Increased secretion of synovial fluid will improve the function of joints.
- Increased hormonal response. One example is glucagon which increases blood glucose levels.

Psychological effects

- Aids mental preparation through visualisation and imagery of the following performance.
- Increases arousal levels – there is an optimum level of arousal which will improve performance but above this level performance will be adversely affected.
- Practise of the activities related to performance may increase confidence.

Examples of warm-up exercises

Warm-up exercises may be selected from the following:

- Alternate heel raising
- Stepping, step-kicks
- Walking around the room
- Brisk walking around the room
- Marching on the spot
- Marching around the room
- Knee bend and grasp with hands
- Skipping

- Alternate leg swinging forwards and backwards
- Alternate leg swinging sideways
- Hip circling
- Pelvic tilting forwards and backwards
- Hip and trunk rotation clockwise and anti-clockwise
- Trunk side bends (caution: keep arms to sides)
- Shoulder shrugging
- Shoulder circling backwards and forwards
- Arm swinging across body, chest press, shoulder press
- Arm circling, beginning with small circles and increasing the range, or upward rowing
- Elbow bending and extending with backward arm swing
- Alternate arm and trunk upward stretch
- Neck flexion, extension (do not hyper extend), side flexion and rotation
- Combine leg and arm movements.

Cool-down/warm-down

This is performed at the end of a performance or exercise session. It reverses the processes that occur during warm-up and allows the body systems to gradually return to a balanced state. Again cool-down is performed for 15–20 minutes. Some of the performance activities can be repeated but at a low level of intensity. Active movements of the large muscle groups of the legs must also be included. The final part will be stretch movements of all the previously used muscles. Rest and deep breathing may be added to finish.

Effects of cool-down

- To keep the heart rate and blood flow elevated. This blood flow will flush the metabolic waste products out of the muscles which will help reduce the pain and stiffness often experienced following exercise.
- To maintain muscle contraction. If the exercises stopped suddenly, the heart is no longer helped by the contracting muscles – this will increase the demand on the cardio-vascular system and heart rate will rise.
- To maintain the pumping action of the contracting muscles to prevent blood pooling in the legs due to the dilation of the blood vessel and the capillaries. This pooling of blood in the legs results in a reduction in blood flow to the brain, which may cause dizziness and fainting.
- Stretching after exercise is important as it has been shown that this also reduces 'delayed onset muscle soreness' (DOMS).

LEARN

Always begin the routine with easy, gentle exercises, progress to the more difficult and then end with gentle exercises

COOL-DOWN EXERCISES

Examples of cool-down exercises

- Continue with some movements, from main activities but at lower intensity and pace.
- Skipping
- Jogging
- Walking
- Stepping
- Knee bends to chest

Complete cool-down with some stretch movements.
- Spinal rotation stretch
- Knee-hug hamstring stretch
- Shoulder rotations
- Gastrocnemius stretch

In prone lying:
- Push-up back extension
- Knee-bend quadriceps stretch

In long sitting
- Gastrocnemius stretch
- Hamstring stretch
- Spinal rotation stretch

End the class with deep breathing in the lying position and get up slowly.

MOBILITY EXERCISES

Neck mobility
Note: keep the shoulders relaxed throughout.

Starting position	Exercise
■ Stride standing or sitting	tuck the chin in and drop the head forwards, then lift the chin and take the head backwards slightly. (Caution: do not hyper-extend.)

■ Stride standing or sitting	looking straight ahead, take the head sideways, the ear towards the shoulder, first to the right and then to the left.
■ Stride standing or sitting	keeping the chin in, turn the head towards the right shoulder and then the left shoulder.
■ Stride standing or sitting	tuck the chin in, drop the head forwards and keep the chin on the chest. Then turn the head to the right and then the left.

Do not circle the head round and round or hyper extend as this can damage the cervical joints and cause pressure on the spinal nerves in this area.

Shoulder mobility

Starting position	Exercise
■ Stride standing or sitting	pull the shoulders back and relax. Lift the shoulders up and down.
■ Stride standing or sitting	circle the shoulders forward, upwards, backwards and down, then the other way.
■ Stride standing	swing the arms forwards and up above the head, then down and backwards.
■ Stride standing	swing the arms sideways and up to cross above the head, then down to cross behind the back.

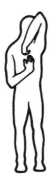

FIGURE NUMBER: 12.1

■ Stride standing	keep the elbows straight and rotate the arms medially and laterally (turn in and out).
■ Stride standing	circle the arms backwards alternately and then together.
■ Stride standing	swing the arms backwards alternately and then together.
■ Stride standing	raise the arms sideways to clap above the head and then lower them to clap the sides.
■ Stride standing	place the right hand behind the neck and the left arm behind the back, trying to touch hands, then change hands.
■ Stride standing or sitting	reach forward, keeping the arms at shoulder level, cross the arms and clasp the hands, lift the arms straight above the head and push backwards behind the head.
■ Yard stride standing	bend the elbows with the palms facing forward, drop the arms so that the palms face backwards and rotate the arms up and down.

Combinations of the above movements can be used and performed to music. Towels, bars and dumb-bells can be used to add variety and interest.

■ Prone kneeling on elbows (not hands)	resting the chin on one hand, take the other arm under the body and stretch it down the outside of opposite leg, then take it out and lift it out to the side. Repeat with the other arm.

Trunk mobility

Starting position	*Exercise*
■ Stride standing, hands on thighs	keeping the chin in, curl the trunk forwards while sliding the hands down the thighs.

■ Stride standing, hands on buttocks

extend the trunk backwards while sliding the hands down the buttocks.

■ Stride standing, hands to sides

bend the trunk to the right and then to the left while sliding the hands down the sides.

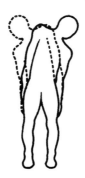

FIGURE NUMBER: 12.2

■ Crook lying

pressing the lower back into the floor, bend alternate legs onto the chest.

■ Crook lying

bend both legs onto the chest.

■ Crook lying

bend both legs onto the chest and lift the head and shoulders towards the knees, clasping the knees with the hands.

■ Crook lying

keep the shoulders against the floor. Tip both knees to the right and then to the left. Keep the knees together.

■ Supine lying

stretch the right arm down the right side and the left arm down the left side.

■ Prone kneeling with back flat

arch the back upwards, pull in the stomach, lower the back and hollow it gently.

■ Prone kneeling with back flat

bend the right knee onto the chest, arch the back and kick out behind. Repeat with the left leg. (Caution: perform this exercise carefully, lifting the leg only fifteen degrees above horizontal.)

■ Prone kneeling	stretch the opposite arm and leg outwards and upwards. Repeat with the other side.
■ Supine lying	lift the right leg to a right angle to the body. Lower the leg towards the floor on the left side of the body, twisting the trunk gently. Repeat with the other leg.
■ Prone lying	lift the opposite arm and leg upwards. Repeat on the other side.

Hip mobility

Starting position	Exercise
■ Support standing	raise one leg and swing it forwards and backwards. Keep the toes pointing forwards, do not move the trunk and keep the hip forwards. Repeat with the other leg.
■ Support standing	raise one leg out sideways and swing it sideways and back across the other leg. Keep the toe pointing forwards and do not move the trunk. Repeat with the other leg.
■ Support standing	raise one leg and circle it around. Repeat with the other leg.
■ Prone kneeling	bend the knee up to the chest and move out and up. Repeat with the other leg. (Caution: this should be performed carefully, lifting the leg only fifteen degrees above horizontal.)
■ Supine lying	part the legs and bring them together.
■ Crook lying	drop the knees outwards and bring them together.

■ Supine lying	bend the knees onto the chest and straighten them into the air, keeping them at 90° to the body. Open and cross the legs in a scissor movement. Bend the knees to the chest to lower them.
■ Standing	run on the spot, lifting the knees higher and higher.
■ Standing	star jumping – jump feet into stride standing position and back. (Caution: do not abduct too far.) Only for the young and agile.
■ Walk standing	bring back foot forwards and take forward foot back by jumping.

Knee mobility

Starting position	*Exercise*
■ High sitting on a chair or the end of a couch	swing the lower legs up and down from bent to straight knee.
■ Prone lying on a couch, with feet over the end	bend alternate knees, bringing heel to buttock, and straighten.
■ Prone lying on a couch, with feet over the end	bend one knee and cross the other leg over the back of the bent leg. Now push with the back leg to increase the bend in the front leg. This is useful if there is limited range in the knee joint. Repeat with the other leg.
■ Supine lying	bend one knee onto the chest. Kick it out straight and lower it. If bending is limited, grasp the knee with hands and pull it into the body. Repeat with the other leg. (Caution: DO NOT perform this exercise with both legs together.)
■ Supine lying	bend the knees onto the chest and straighten them into the air. Cycle the legs in the air.

■ Support standing	hold onto a wall bar with the hands at shoulder height. Bend the knees and hips down to the squatting position, hold and straighten. (Caution: do not take the buttocks below the knees.) Only for young and agile.

Foot mobility

Starting position	*Exercise*
■ Sitting with feet on floor	■ push the toes into the floor (do not let them curl); ■ raise the toes away from the floor; ■ spread the toes outwards and together; ■ move the big toes towards each other; ■ pick up a pencil with the toes.
■ Sitting with feet on floor and a towel or strap lengthways under foot	Keeping the heel firmly pressed onto towel, use the toes to pull the towel towards the heel.
■ Sitting with feet on floor and a towel or strap widthways under foot	Keeping the heel on the ground, move the towel to one side and then the other.
■ Sitting with hands over top of toes	push down with the hand and lift the toes up against the resistance.
■ Sitting with hands under the toes	push up with the hand and push down with the toes against the resistance.
■ Sitting with one leg across the other at the knee	turn the foot in and out.
■ Sitting with one leg across the other at the knee	pull the foot up and down.
■ Sitting with one leg across the other at the knee	circle the foot ten times one way and ten times the opposite way.
■ Long sitting	turn the feet inwards and press the inner arches together.

Additional exercises:

- Walk around, moving the weight from the heel to the outer border to the ball of the foot.
- Walk in a straight line, moving the weight from the heel to the outer border to the ball of the foot.
- Walk around on the toes.
- Walk around on the heels.
- Walk normally.
- Skip or jog, changing direction.
- Hop on one leg, then the other (only for young and agile).
- Jump forwards, backwards and sideways.
- Jump to stride and back, jump to walk and back.

TASK

Work as a group. Each member of the group must devise and teach five mobility exercises for one named joint. Each person should take a different joint.

THE BENEFITS OF EXERCISE

Research has shown that regular exercise is beneficial for all age groups. We have seen from our study of the body systems how they make physiological adaptations in response to exercise or overload. The extent of these changes will depend on the type of exercise and on the systems subjected to stress. Appropriate exercises regularly practised will improve physical fitness, promote health and reduce the risk of developing many diseases. Even moderate activities will improve health and the quality of life. Activities need not be specific exercise. Gardening, walking, vacuuming, dancing or any activity which expends energy will result in improvement providing it is done for 30 mins, 5–6 times/week. The greater the energy expenditure the greater the benefits. The beneficial effects derived from exercise are both physiological and psychological.

Physiological benefits:

- improvement in cardio-vascular function, i.e. heart and circulation;
- improvement in respiratory function, i.e. lungs and breathing;
- improvement in muscle tone, strength and stamina, which in turn improves posture and body contours (shape);
- improvement in the flexibility and tensile strength of tendons and ligaments. This will increase the range of movement at joints and reduce the likelihood of trauma;
- improvement in the condition of joints. Exercise increases the production of synovial fluid, which lubricates and nourishes the cartilage;
- improvement in bone density, which will combat osteoporosis;
- improvement in neuro-muscular co-ordination, which improves skills such as rhythm, balance, timing, reaction time and co-ordination;

- increase in metabolic rate, with reduction in fat reserves. Muscle tissue has a high metabolic rate, therefore the more muscle tissue on the body, the higher the metabolic rate. This will increase demand for fuel and thus reduce fat stores;
- lowering of blood cholesterol levels;
- reduction in trauma and pain due to improved posture, strength and flexibility.

The psychological benefits are:
- feelings of well-being, achievement and euphoria;
- an increase in self-confidence and self-esteem;
- reduction in stress levels;
- promotion of relaxation and sleep.

Health-related benefits
- Reduces the risk of developing high blood pressure.
- Helps to reduce high blood pressure in those who suffer from it.
- Reduces the risk of developing heart disease.
- Reduces the risk of developing diabetes.
- Reduces the risk of developing vascular disease such as atherosclerosis (which is narrowing and hardening of the arteries, caused by the build up of fatty plaques on the vessel walls).
- Helps to reduce body weight and improve body shape.
- Helps to reduce cholesterol levels.
- Reduces the risk of developing colon cancer.
- Helps to build stronger bones thus reducing the risk of developing osteoporosis.
- Helps to prevent joint problems.
- Maintains strength and mobility therefore improving quality of life.
- Reduces anxiety and depression.

To achieve these benefits, exercises must be carefully selected and accurately and carefully performed. Exercise should always be specific to the individual, and the degree of ease or difficulty should be appropriate for the level of fitness. Inappropriate exercises that are too difficult or are casually and excessively performed can result in damage and pain.

Damaging effects of inappropriate exercise
- muscle strain, tears and soreness;
- ligamentous sprains, overstretching and tears;
- joint stresses;
- bone stresses;
- inflammation of tendons, bursae and joint capsules, namely tendonitis, bursitis and capsulitis;
- pain, which adversely affects daily activities, relaxation and sleep. Pain may also produce feelings of tension, stress, depression, disappointment and low self-esteem.

IMPORTANT POINTS TO REMEMBER

- To improve fitness, the principle of overload and progression must be applied. The intensity of exercise must be greater than that normally encountered and must become progressively harder. Repeating the same exercise a set number of times will maintain a level of fitness but will not result in significant improvement. The variables that are used to increase overload are *intensity*, *duration* and *frequency*.

- Different types of exercise stress different body systems and produce different effects. Cardio-respiratory or aerobic endurance is a fundamental requirement of fitness for everyone. Other components should be specific to the sport or performance and meet the needs of the individual.

- Muscle flexibility and the range of joint movement will improve through regular stretching exercises.

- Muscle strength and bulk will increase through strengthening exercises, i.e. regularly working the muscle against progressive resistance. The degree of tension developed in a muscle will be directly proportional to the overload. Fewer repetitions at maximum overload will increase muscle strength.

- Muscle endurance, i.e. the capacity of a muscle to repeat an activity without fatigue, will improve if the muscle is made to perform repetitive movements. High repetitions with low resistance will increase muscle endurance.

- Speed will increase if movements and activities are practised at increasing pace.

- Skill, agility, balance and co-ordination develop through repeated practice of an activity, increasing the difficulty by altering the base, the centre of gravity and the pace.

- Cardio-respiratory endurance will improve in response to regular practice of aerobic activities such as jogging, walking, cycling, swimming and aerobic exercise classes. The exercises must be slow and steady and increase very gradually in intensity. This allows the heart, blood vessels and lungs to deliver sufficient oxygen to the muscles for the complete breakdown of glycogen. If the exercises become too fast or intense, then anaerobic metabolism takes over.

- To deliver aerobic endurance, the heart rate must be raised, but it must not be raised beyond 80–90 per cent of an individual's maximum heart rate. Remember: MHR is calculated as 220 minus the person's age. Initially, the pulse rate should be raised to only 60 per cent of MHR, progressing to 70 per cent and then to 80–90 per cent. The elevated heart rate must be maintained for fifteen to twenty minutes per session. Exercise should be repeated three to four times per week on alternate days to allow time for recovery.

- To develop anaerobic systems, short sharp bursts of activity must be practised. These should be explosive and dynamic activities such as squash, fast sprints, shot putting, etc.

- Spot reduction of fat through exercise is *not* possible. Exercising a specific area of the body will improve muscle tone in that area, but will not disperse covering fat. To reduce body fat, calories consumed (intake) must be less than calories used (output). Only then is fat removed from all over the body and broken down for energy. Long duration aerobic exercises are high calorie burners, use fat for energy and are the best way of reducing body fat. Strengthening exercises are low calorie burners, so lots of curl-ups will not remove fat from the abdomen, although they will improve the strength of abdominal muscles.

■ Weight is often gained rather than lost when people take up exercise, even though fat is reduced. This is because muscle tissue is heavier than fat. Losing weight is not an indication of fitness: it is the ratio of fat to fat-free tissue that is important. More muscle and less fat will result in an increase in fitness and better body shape.

■ Muscle tissue has a high metabolic rate. Therefore having more muscle tissue gives an individual a higher metabolic rate, which means that calories are burnt up more quickly. This makes it easier to lose weight. Through regular exercise people who burn calories slowly can become high calorie burners, thus reducing fat stores more rapidly.

■ Muscles will not change to fat if exercising stops, as is commonly supposed. However, muscle strength will be reduced and the muscles will feel softer. Muscle and fat are completely different tissues. Fat is stored on the body as a reserve of energy if calorific intake is greater than calorific output.

■ The warm-up is a very important part of all training and exercise routines. It enables the energy systems to increase their rate of work gradually. It warms muscles, which improves their contractability and flexibility. It improves the flexibility of connective tissue components and reduces the likelihood of injury. The warm-up should include mobilising exercises, pulse-raising exercises and simple static stretch.

■ The cool-down or warm-down is equally important, as it allows the system to slow down gradually and aids the removal of the waste products lactic acid and carbon dioxide. The cool-down enables the body to return to a stable state, i.e. homeostasis is re-established. Cool-down will include less strenuous or gentle activity and stretching of the muscles used in the training.

■ Exercises should never stop suddenly, nor should one stand still after vigorous exercise, as fainting and dizziness may result. During vigorous exercise the blood vessels supplying the muscles dilate, which increases the load on the heart, but the contracting muscles assist in pumping the blood around the body. If exercise stops suddenly, the vessels are still dilated and blood pools in the legs due to gravitational pull. This deprives the brain of oxygen, causing dizziness and faintness. The pressure on the heart is increased as it attempts to maintain blood supply. The cool-down must include gentle activity such as jogging or walking around, followed by stretching and breathing exercises that are performed while lying down.

Exercise and asthma

Asthma sufferers may exercise with caution, but must not over-exert. One must always bear in mind that physical exertion can sometimes trigger an asthmatic attack. This is referred to as exercise-induced asthma. If breathing difficulties are experienced for longer than normal, i.e. over five minutes, and there is obvious distress, then medical advice should be sought quickly. Asthmatics should always have bronchodilators to hand, and must learn to recognise distress signals and take appropriate steps to control the condition.

Chapter 13
Safety and hygiene factors related to exercise

SAFETY

The safety of clients and other staff is of paramount importance and is the responsibility of the therapist in charge. Every precaution should be taken to create conditions and consider factors which will avoid injury.

The factors which contribute to injuries are:
- Inadequate demonstration, unclear commands or poor tuition.
- Activities that are too difficult and inappropriate to age and fitness levels.
- Excessive overload or too rapid an increase of overload.
- Failure to warm-up and cool-down adequately.
- Inadequate rest during the exercise session.
- Inadequate recovery time between sessions.
- Ignoring contra-indications and proceeding with exercise.
- Ignoring signs of stress while exercising and not stopping.
- Incomplete recovery from previous injury.
- Faulty equipment.
- Improper use of equipment.

- Equipment left lying around in the working area.
- Insufficient space and overcrowding.
- Inappropriate footwear and clothing.
- Intensive competition among participants.
- Poor exercise technique and poor body alignment.
- Inappropriate starting positions.
- Performing potentially damaging exercises.
- Dehydration.

This is a long list but you may be able to think of other factors. The following guidelines will help you to take the precautions necessary to avoid injury.

CONTRA-INDICATIONS TO EXERCISE

All clients should have a thorough consultation before embarking on an exercise programme. Any of the following conditions would indicate that the client should not exercise. Unfamiliar conditions may be highlighted during consultation. If in doubt, always seek medical advice.

Common contra-indications are:
- *any recent injuries:* these would include fractures, strains, sprains, ruptures or tears. It is sometimes desirable to maintain fitness in other parts of the body while the injured part is immobilised. The exercises for other body parts must be carefully planned and performed, ensuring that no stress is placed on the injured part and surrounding tissues;
- *heart conditions* or any history of heart disease. Appropriate exercise regimes are undertaken following heart attacks and surgery, but these should be medically directed or supervised;
- *high blood pressure:* generally, if the blood pressure is controlled by drugs, exercise is allowed, but check with the client's doctor. Relaxation can help hypertensive clients, but isometrics should never be performed;
- *any acute fevers,* such as influenza, glandular fever, the common cold, etc;
- *any infections,* such as throat infections, measles, chicken pox, etc;
- *any inflammatory joint conditions,* such as arthritis. Rheumatoid arthritis is a systemic condition in which joints become hot, swollen and stiff. Osteoarthritis is a condition of wear of the joints, the cartilage wears thin, making movement very painful;
- *neurological disorders,* such as strokes, multiple sclerosis, etc. – exercises for these conditions must be medically supervised;
- *undiagnosed illness:* seek a doctor's advice;
- *musculo-skeletal problems,* such as joint or back pain;
- *pain and soreness in muscles* caused by trauma or injury as opposed to delayed onset of muscle stiffness;
- *pregnancy,* medical consent must be sought and gentle exercises only should be given. During the first three months of pregnancy, particular care must be taken. The fit client

who has exercised regularly may continue with low-impact, low-intensity work. Weights should not be used, nor should exercises that increase intra-abdominal pressure be performed.

■ after eating a *heavy meal* or under the influence of alcohol;
■ if *overtired* or exhausted;
■ if under the influence of *pain-killing* drugs;
■ if there has been any *past difficulty* with exercise.
■ Diabetics must obtain medical advice and approval. Low or moderate intensity exercise is normally recommended.

Be particularly aware of increasing problems with age. To be safe, all those over 40 should have a medical check-up before starting an exercise programme.

Those who are at greatest risk are:
■ obese people;
■ those with a history of heart problems in the immediate family;
■ hypertensives;
■ diabetics – a doctor's referral is important, especially if the client is on insulin;
■ those with a history of lung problems, such as asthma, bronchitis or emphysema;
■ smokers.

Refer these people for a check-up before commencing exercise programmes.

SAFETY FACTORS TO OBSERVE WHILE EXERCISING

The premises
■ The room should be warm, well ventilated and without draughts. It must not be too hot.
■ There must be good, even lighting, with no pools of light or dark corners.
■ Lights should be shielded with guards, particularly if games are played.
■ The floor should be firm, smooth and non-slip, and preferably sprung.
■ There must be sufficient space for everyone to move freely, with no overcrowding.
■ The room should be clean and uncluttered; all apparatus not in use should be stored neatly away from the working area.
■ Apparatus should be in good condition; there should be no rough edges or sharp protruding parts that could cause injury.
■ There must be a sufficient number of well-marked fire exits.
■ A well-stocked first-aid box should be clearly visible and accessible.
■ Shower and toilet facilities should be available.
■ Drinking water should be available but kept away from the working area.

- Water and fluids must be kept away from the working area, as spillages make the floor slippery and dangerous.
- There should be no eating or drinking in the working area.
- Exercises should be supervised by qualified instructors at all times. Accurate demonstration and instruction must be given.
- Protective mats should be available for floor exercises, one per client.
- Mirrors should be available to check body alignment and to correct the performance of activities.

The client

- Suitable clothing that will allow free, unrestricted movement must be worn. Cotton is the best fabric, as it allows easy absorption of perspiration. Cotton vests or T-shirts and shorts with elasticated waists, or cotton bodies, are all suitable.

  Some athletes wear track suits and leg-warmers to maintain or raise body temperature during the warm-up and stretch routines.
- Footwear must be chosen with care to suit the activity. Well-constructed shoes should be bought from a reputable manufacturer. Footwear for exercise should be light and comfortable and offer good lateral support. The toe box should have sufficient height, breadth and length to prevent the toes rubbing. The inner sole should absorb shock and the outer sole should be pliable, durable and non-slip. The tongue should be padded to protect the dorsum of the foot and the heel tab should not be too high and should not press on the heel.

  Socks alone should never be used for exercise because of the danger of slipping, but they should be worn with shoes to reduce friction.
- Hair should be tied back off the face. Hair combs, slides and pins should be avoided.
- Jewellery should be removed.
- Check for contra-indications: if in doubt, seek a doctor's advice.
- Clients must not exercise after a heavy meal, nor under the influence of alcohol. Allow at least two hours after eating.
- Clients must not exercise if pain-killing drugs have been taken.
- All equipment to be used must be fully demonstrated, its effect explained and safety factors highlighted.
- Exercise or training must be specific to the individual. Clients must work at their own pace and level, must not exceed their target rate
- Clients should not be encouraged or allowed to compete against each other
- The different levels of fitness and the age range of those present must always be carefully considered when giving group exercise. Individuals must rest when tired and must not exceed their maximum heart rate during performance.
- Exercises should not cause pain – clients must be advised to stop exercising if pain is experienced.
- Select safe, stable starting positions.
- Exercises must be clearly explained and demonstrated accurately and any precautions must be stressed. The client must fully understand the exercise and be aware of potential hazards.

- Ensure that good posture and body alignment are maintained when exercises are performed to prevent stresses and strains.
- Teach the client the correct breathing patterns. They must not hold their breath.
- Ensure that the clients perform a thorough warm-up lasting ten to fifteen minutes that includes all the large muscle groups.
- Ensure that clients stretch carefully, slowly and smoothly, and include all the main joints. After the main activity, make sure that clients perform a cool-down (warm-down). Stretch again, then finish with relaxation and deep breathing.
- Ensure that the clients perform adequate cool-down.
- Ensure that clients do not stop exercising suddenly.

Remember:
- Do not exercise or stretch cold muscles.
- Always practise warm-up exercises.
- Warming the tissues with various forms of heat therapy and massage will help, but it is not enough; warm-up exercises must be done, as they allow the body systems to build up gradually to meet the demand placed on them. Include mobilisers, pulse raisers and simple stretches.
- Increase to peak intensity very gradually and decrease gradually.

GUIDELINES FOR EXERCISE

These can be displayed in the exercise room or fully explained to clients at the beginning of the course.

Considerations before you start

- Wear suitable clothing and well-fitting shoes and socks.
- Do not exercise in socks.
- Tie your hair back off the face with ribbons or bands.
- Remove all jewellery except rings.
- Check the list of contra-indications. Do not exercise if you know or suspect that you are affected by any on the list.
- If you are suffering from any other illness, please report it. Check with your doctor whether exercising is suitable.
- Do not exercise after a heavy meal: allow at least two hours to elapse.
- Do not exercise if under the influence of alcohol or pain-killing drugs.
- Do not exercise if you are feeling tired and fatigued, nor if suffering from muscle soreness except delayed onset of muscle soreness following other activities, in which case exercise carefully.
- Empty the bladder before exercise.
- Complete the Client Record Card and sign the consent form.

Considerations during and after exercise

■ Do not strain. Exercise should not produce pain.

■ Always work at your own pace. Rest when necessary. Do not compete with others.

■ Calculate your target rate. Take your pulse rate at regular intervals and do not exceed the maximum heart rate for your age. If you are unsure how to do this ask the instructor for help.

■ Keep to a few repetitions at the beginning of the course and add three to five with each session.

■ Do not exercise or stretch cold muscles. Always perform a ten to fifteen minute warm-up first. If you are late for the class, do not join in until you have completed the warm-up.

■ Watch and listen carefully to the instruction. If unsure of detail, ask for help.

■ Learn to perform the exercises correctly. Pay attention to detail.

■ Always exercise carefully, paying full attention throughout. Do no exercise half-heartedly, mechanically or without concentration. Movements should be smooth and co-ordinated.

■ Maintain correct, balanced posture throughout.

■ Stretch carefully, smoothly and slowly, feeling the stretch in the belly of the muscle and not at the tendon ends. Hold the stretch and release slowly.

■ Do not bounce at the end of the muscle range or stretch muscles rapidly. This type of ballistic movement works against the stretch reflex and may result in small tears within the muscle.

■ Breathe freely during exercise. Do not hold the breath when stretching; exhale as you move into the stretch and effort.

■ Maintain good body alignment (posture) while exercising. Avoid strain on vulnerable areas such as the neck, lower back and knees.

■ If injury occurs, stop exercising immediately. Follow the 'RICED' principle to deal with injury – rest, ice, compression, elevation and diagnosis.

■ Drink water at the end of the session to maintain fluid levels.

THE PROGRESSION OF EXERCISE

Progression is essential to maintain and improve the beneficial effects of exercise. The work must be progressively increased in order to maintain overload. There are various ways of making exercises more difficult:

■ increase the frequency, i.e. the number of times an exercise is performed. Begin with six repetitions, then ten, fifteen and twenty. If muscle endurance is the objective, increase the repetitions to 30–50;

■ increase the intensity, i.e. make the muscles work harder by increasing the resistance. Weights, springs, pulley systems, multigyms, etc., are used to provide resistance; change the leverage: begin with a short weight arm and increase the length when the work becomes easy. The leg and arm can be shortened by bending the knee and elbow.

Progression is achieved by straightening the limb, then holding a pole or dumb-bells. The leverage of curl-ups is increased by moving the arm position from the side to across the chest, then putting the hands on the shoulders, etc. Leverage and weight can be combined for progression.

■ Increase the number of sessions, e.g. from twice to three times per week or more. Ensure that there is sufficient rest time for the body to recover fully, otherwise there is risk of damage.

■ To improve cardio-respiratory endurance, increase the duration of the exercise, i.e. the time of each session and/or the length of the training programme.

■ Reduce the stability of the starting position. Exercising becomes more difficult as the starting position becomes less stable. This will improve the skill components of balance, co-ordination and agility.

■ Change the speed at which an exercise is performed. Exercises are easier at natural speed, which varies with the individual. Exercises become more difficult if the speed is increased or decreased.

POTENTIALLY DAMAGING EXERCISES THAT SHOULD BE AVOIDED

There are a number of exercises that produce excessive stress on vulnerable areas of the body, such as the neck, the lower back and the knees, and that may result in injury. Many of these exercises form part of certain training programmes and routines for specific sports. When they are performed by very fit trained athletes in controlled situations the risk of injury is greatly reduced. They should not be performed by unfit individuals, nor included in general exercise or group exercises where individual supervision and control is impossible. The ability to evaluate the safety and effectiveness of an exercise is an important part of an instructor's role. All exercise videos, exercise books and magazine articles should be carefully studied, and each exercise must be analysed and checked for safety, as many of these hazardous exercises are often included. New forms of exercise routines or 'crazes' require particular caution. Because the human body is designed to perform a certain finite number of movements through specific ranges, the so-called 'new' exercises must be versions of the old. Claims made for the results are often exaggerated, and so must be carefully assessed: are they realistic and achievable?

When assessing the safety and effectiveness of an exercise it is useful to ask the following questions:

1 Will the exercise work the appropriate body part?
2 Will the exercise move the selected muscle and joint through the correct range?
3 Will the movement be a controlled, free movement, not forced or ballistic?
4 Is the exercise appropriate for the client's level of fitness?
5 Could the exercise over-stress the moving joints or other body parts, causing damage?
6 Is this the most suitable exercise for achieving the set goal?

7 Will the exercise or the starting position put stress on any of the following vulnerable areas: the cervical region (the neck); the lumbar region (the lower back); the knees?

The following section deals with vulnerable areas of the body, potentially damaging exercises are highlighted and safe alternatives are given where possible.

The seven vertebrae of the cervical region

This is the region of greatest spinal mobility. The first two cervical vertebrae – the atlas and axis – allow rotation of the head. The normal movements of the cervical region are:

- *flexion* – dropping the head forward, chin on chest;
- *extension* – tilting the head backwards – and hyper-extension – taking it beyond extension to look at the ceiling;
- *side flexion* (lateral flexion) – dropping the head sideways, ear towards shoulder;
- *rotation* – turning the head to the right and left, looking towards the shoulder;
- *circumduction* – a combination of the above;

Movements of the chin also affect the cervical region;

- *protraction* of the chin – pushing the chin forward;
- *retraction* of the chin – pulling the chin back and in.

Before commencing exercises for the cervical spine, select a stable starting position such as sitting or stride standing. If the client is very tense, the lying position can be used. Make sure the head is in a good position: erect, with ear lobes level, eyes looking straight ahead and shoulders relaxed.

SAFE EXERCISES

Starting position	Exercise
■ Sitting	drop chin onto chest, return to upright position.
■ Sitting	take right ear down towards right shoulder and back, then left ear towards left shoulder and back.
■ Sitting	turn the head to the right to look towards the right shoulder, repeat to left.

For all these exercises, it is important to keep the chin in and the head up.

DAMAGING EXERCISES
NOT RECOMMENDED

■ Sitting

hyper-extension – dropping the head back to look at the ceiling.

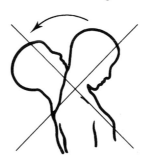

FIGURE NUMBER: 13.1

■ Sitting

circling head around on the shoulders.

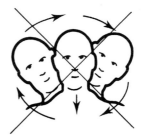

FIGURE NUMBER: 13.2

These two exercises are not recommended as they produce excessive pressure and compression of the cervical discs. These may rupture and protrude into the inter-vertebral foramina, resulting in pressure on and damage to the nerves. This will cause pain, numbness and pins and needles over the shoulder and down the arm.

With age the cervical region is susceptible to wear and tear, with erosion of the cartilage and bone. This may result in inflammation of surrounding structures, with pain and stiffness of the neck. These exercises will exacerbate this condition. They should not be done in general exercise classes, by those over 30 years old or by anyone suffering from headaches, neck pain or shoulder and arm pain, numbness or pins and needles.

DAMAGING EXERCISES
NOT RECOMMENDED

■ Lying

lift legs and lower back upwards and touch the floor behind the head with the toes (the 'plough').

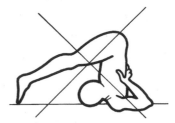

FIGURE NUMBER: 13.3

■ Lying

lift legs and hips off the floor and support with hands, cycle or open/close legs in the air.

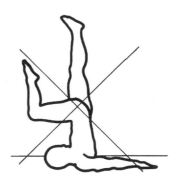

FIGURE NUMBER: 13.4

With both these exercises, the body weight is supported across the shoulders and neck. This imposes severe compression forces on the neck, which can cause damage to ligaments, bones, discs and nerves. This position also compresses the chest, thus reducing the working and efficiency of the heart and lungs.

The five vertebrae of the lumbar region

The lower back is a vulnerable area because it supports the whole weight of the upper body before it is distributed to the pelvis. The movements of the lumbar region are:

■ *flexion* – bending forward;
■ *extension* – moving the trunk backwards;
■ limited *side flexion* – bending to the side;
■ negligible *rotation* – turning the trunk right and left is negligible in the lumbar region; most trunk rotation occurs in the thoracic region.

The lumbar region is where most trunk flexion occurs. It is the fulcrum for this movement, where the weight is the upper trunk and the weight arm is the length of the trunk moving about the fulcrum. The effort is supplied by the back extensors and the effort arm is the distance of their insertion from the fulcrum.

Considerable stress is placed on the lumbar spine during forward flexion and the return to extension. The amount of stress is influenced by two factors:
1 the length of the weight arm and the amount of weight;
2 the degree of rotation of the pelvis that accompanies the movement.

The trunk extensors (the erector spinae) and the antagonistic trunk flexors (the abdominals) must be strong and balanced to support the trunk and maintain the stability of the pelvis. Imbalance between these muscles alters the pelvic tilt and imposes stresses on the lumbar spine.
- Weakness of the abdominals results in forward pelvic tilt and lordosis of the lumbar spine.
- Weakness of the erector spinae results in backward pelvic tilt and flat back.

SAFE EXERCISE

■ Stride standing, hands on legs (knees soft)	slowly bend forwards, sliding the hands down the legs, then return to upright position.

Particular care must be taken when straightening up: always rotate the pelvis backwards first and then extend the lumbar spine. The instruction to clients on returning to the upright position should be
- pull their bottom in and straighten inch by inch from the bottom of the spine upwards.

DAMAGING EXERCISES
NOT RECOMMENDED

■ Stretch, stride standing	bend forward to touch floor and swing up.

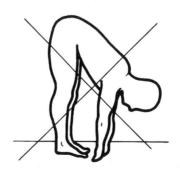

FIGURE NUMBER: 13.5

■ Stretch, stride standing

bend to touch opposite foot with hand.

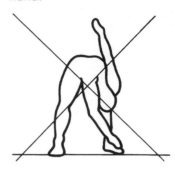

FIGURE NUMBER: 13.6

■ Stride standing holding a pole across back of shoulders

Twist right and left.

In these positions, with the arms stretched above the head, the weight arm is lengthened and there is a far greater load in front of the fulcrum (the lumbar spine). This increases the stress and compression on the discs, and damage can occur to ligaments, discs, cartilage or bones.

Punching the air with the hands in forward flexion imposes the same stress and is not recommended. Rotating the trunk to touch the opposite foot increases the compression forces still further.

Ballistic-type bouncing at the end of the range of forward flexion in order to stretch the hamstrings must be avoided. This exerts excessive pressure on the lower back and may produce microtears and damage to the hamstrings. Since the hamstrings are not relaxed in this position but are contracting eccentrically, stretching is ineffective and can cause damage.

SAFE EXERCISE

■ Stride standing

trunk side flexion to the right and left, slide hand down side.

The same principle of leverage applies to this exercise, which will be safe if the arms are kept down to the side, keeping the weight arm as short as possible.

DAMAGING EXERCISES
NOT RECOMMENDED

■ Stride standing

swing left arm into the air and side flex laterally to the right, then return and swing right arm up and side flex laterally to the left.

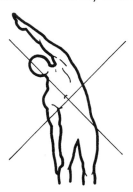

FIGURE NUMBER: 13.7

The arm is stretched up into the air, increasing the length of the weight arm. The increased leverage imposes stresses on the lumbar joints and discs, causing damage. Again, ballistic bounding at the end of the range will make the exercise even more hazardous.

DAMAGING EXERCISES
NOT RECOMMENDED

■ Side lying

lift both legs upwards.

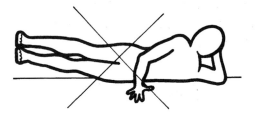

FIGURE NUMBER: 13.8

The trunk side flexors will strain to lift the legs. This stresses the lower back. Twisting of the trunk while straining to lift the legs causes further damage.

Abdominal strengthening exercises

SAFE EXERCISES

■ Crook lying	press small of back into floor, tilt pelvis backwards and pull in the abdominals.
■ Crook lying, hands across chest	curl up head towards knees.
■ Crook lying	raise bent knees towards ceiling.

The second exercise can be safely progressed by moving the arm position, thus lengthening the weight arm: for example with the hands on the shoulders, the hands beside the head, the hands stretched above the head. (The hands should not, however, be clasped behind the head, as this can stress and damage the neck; instead, place the hands beside the head above the ears.)

The exercise can be progressed further by holding a weight across the chest and above the head.

DAMAGING EXERCISES
NOT RECOMMENDED

■ Lying	double leg raising.

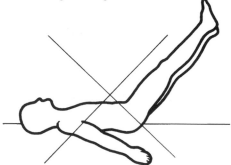

FIGURE NUMBER: 13.9

■ Lying	straight leg sit-ups.

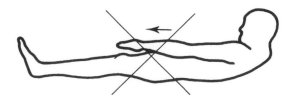

FIGURE NUMBER: 13.10

■ Crook lying	Twist sit ups.

Both these exercises impose stress and can cause many problems. They are not effective in strengthening the abdominal muscles, as can be seen by analysing the movement.

Moving joint:	hip joint
Direction of movement:	flexion coming up, extension going down
Prime movers:	ilio-psoas (hip flexor)
Muscle work:	concentric coming up, eccentric going down.

The psoas is a short muscle passing from the lumbar vertebrae to the lesser trochanter of the femur. It works with the iliacus and both muscles may be named ilio-psoas. As the psoas lifts the legs or the trunk it pulls on its origin on the lumbar spine, imposing stresses and strains in this region. The psoas is working at tremendous mechanical disadvantage, as it is made to lift a long weight arm with a large weight (that of the legs). The back arches and strain is felt in the lumbar spine.

With this exercise, the psoas becomes stronger and tighter. This is undesirable, because a tight posas pulls and tilts the pelvis forwards, resulting in lordosis due to muscle imbalance.

The abdominal muscles will be working statically in outer range in an attempt to keep the pelvis level. This type of muscle work is extremely difficult to maintain and can only be done by very strong muscles; weaker muscles will be strained.

Static work of the abdominals increases intra-abdominal pressure, which will push on the pelvic organs and stretch the pelvic floor. The muscles of the pelvic floor may already be weakened in post-natal women and older age groups. Strength must be maintained in the pelvic floor to prevent incontinence.

Back strengthening exercises

SAFE EXERCISES

■ Prone lying	alternate single leg raising.
■ Prone lying	alternate arm raising.
■ Prone lying	opposite arm and leg raising.

DAMAGING EXERCISES
NOT RECOMMENDED

■ Prone lying   double leg raising.

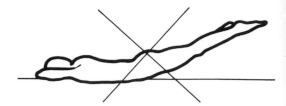

FIGURE NUMBER: 13.11

■ Prone lying   double leg, arm and trunk raising.

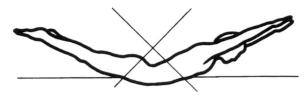

FIGURE NUMBER: 13.12

■ Prone lying   trunk extension, touching feet with hands.

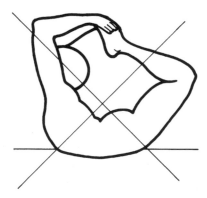

FIGURE NUMBER: 13.13

Raising both legs or, worse, raising both legs and arms, imposes severe compression and stress on the lumbar spine.

Gluteal strengthening exercises

SAFE EXERCISES

■ Prone lying	raise alternate legs off the floor and lower (keep hips in contact with the floor and raise legs only fifteen degrees from floor).
■ Prone kneeling	straighten alternate legs backwards (lifting no more than fifteen degrees from horizontal) and lower.

NOT RECOMMENDED

■ Prone kneeling	bend knee onto chest and kick out behind.

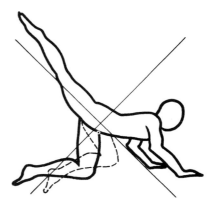

FIGURE NUMBER: 13.14

Raising the leg more than fifteen degrees above the horizontal can stress the lumbar spine. Also, this exercise uses the hip flexor (ilio-psoas) to bend the knee towards the chest (this does not usually require strengthening). This exercise is frequently performed in a swinging manner, where the movement is not controlled and is likely to cause damage.

The knee joint

The stability of the knee is maintained by several strong ligaments (the medial and lateral ligaments and the cruciate ligaments), by powerful muscles (the quadriceps and hamstrings) and by the fascia of the high (the fascia lata).

The movements of the knee are:
■ *flexion* – bending the knee;
■ *extension* – straightening the knee;
■ a slight amount of *rotation* in flexion.

SAFE EXERCISE

■ Long sitting

bend right knee and rotate hip outwards, drop knee onto floor and place foot against left thigh. Place hands on either side of left leg and gently slide hands down left leg forwards. Repeat on opposite side.

DAMAGING EXERCISES
NOT RECOMMENDED

■ Long sitting

bend right knee, turn leg backwards, slide hands along left leg to touch toes (hurdler's stretch).

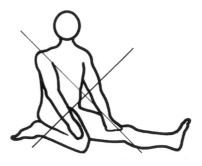

FIGURE NUMBER: 13.15

■ Long sitting

forward flexion, bringing head down onto knees.

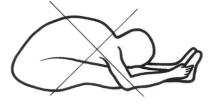

FIGURE NUMBER: 13.16

■ Standing

one leg propped up at right angles, bend forwards sliding hands down leg.

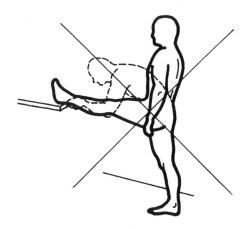

FIGURE NUMBER: 13.17

The flexion of the knee backwards in the hurdler's stretch stresses the medial ligaments of the knee. This method also stresses the lower back, as excessive forward flexion stresses the back.

SAFE EXERCISE

■ Standing, stride or walk standing	bend knees until they are at 90°, bend. Do not allow buttocks to go below the knees. Keep back straight.

DAMAGING EXERCISES
NOT RECOMMENDED

■ Standing, stride or walk standing	bend or squat beyond 90°, allowing the buttocks to go below the knees, and with flexion of trunk.

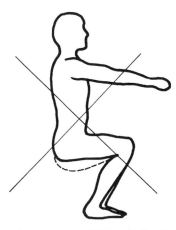

FIGURE NUMBER: 13.18

■ Standing

squatting then jumping and
stretching leg out to side.

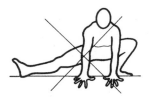

FIGURE NUMBER: 13.19

Squatting and bending the knees beyond 90° while they are supporting the body weight can impose severe stress on the knee joint.

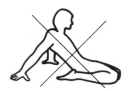

FIGURE NUMBER: 13.20

'Heel sitting' should be avoided by all except the young and very fit, as it stresses and can damage the knee joint. In this position the weight of the body pulls the knee joint open, and this can damage the cartilage and strain the ligaments.

Kneeling and modifications of kneeling should not be used as a starting position for the older client, nor for anyone with knee pain.

Damaging exercises that should be avoided
■ Double leg raising or sit-ups with straight legs or full sit-ups
■ Twist sit-ups
■ Hurdler's stretch, either standing or long sitting
■ Pliés
■ Deep squats
■ Forward flexion where the trunk is at 90° to the legs
■ The 'plough' (resting on head and shoulders with the legs in the air)
■ Head circling
■ Head hyper-extension
■ Very wide 'jumping jacks' with the knees opening wider than the toes: keep the knees in line with the toes
■ Any ballistics, i.e. bouncing at the end of range in stretches such as toe touching, side bending, trunk twisting

- Moving from heel sitting up to kneeling, except for the young and athletic (i.e. those with strong quadriceps). It should not be performed by anyone with knee problems nor those over 50. The same applies to exercises using kneeling as a starting position.
- Back hyper-extension.
- Vigorous kickback in prone kneeling
- Hyper extending spine in crook lying for gluteal strength
- Deep lunges
- Stride standing holding pole behind shoulder trunk twist.

TASK

Work with a partner.
- Teach your partner safe head and neck movements.
- Teach your partner safe trunk forward flexion, side flexion and back extension exercises.
- Explain why the following movements should not be performed:
  a head circling and hyper-extension
  b double leg raising and straight leg sit-ups
  c deep squatting with the bottom lower than the knees.

CLIENT ASSESSMENT

The assessment of a client prior to exercise has developed considerably over the last few years. In addition to obtaining information regarding health, medical history and taking measurements of height, weight, fat distribution and muscle tone, it is now desirable to assess fitness by measuring the pulse rate, blood pressure, lung capacity, muscle strength, muscle endurance, flexibility and body composition.

Accurate assessment is important for the following reasons:
- It provides information on the client's past and present state of health. This will highlight any contra-indications or any conditions where caution is necessary.
- It provides information on the client's lifestyle, activities, athleticism and motivation.
- It establishes the figure type, i.e. endomorph, ectomorph or mesomorph. This facilitates the planning and setting of realistic, achievable goals.
- It identifies postural problems and muscle imbalance, so that specific strategies to restore balance can be planned.
- It establishes the current level of fitness, which provides a starting point for the exercise programme.
- It provides the information necessary for setting objectives and planning safe, effective exercise that will not place the client at risk.
- It provides a record of data and the starting point from which future improvement can be measured.

Preparation of the client prior to fitness assessment

Advise the client:

- to wear comfortable, loose-fitting clothes;
- not to eat for two to three hours before the test;
- not to smoke before or during the test;
- not to drink tea or coffee before the test;
- to empty the bladder before the test;
- to avoid other exercises before the test;
- to concentrate fully on the test;
- to say immediately if they do not understand the instructions and what is required of them.

Height measurement

Method:

- Instruct the client to stand in bare feet with feet together and the back against the measure. Ask the client to stand straight and look directly ahead.
- Bring the measure bar down so that it just touches the head, read the measurement, record it on the client's card and inform the client.

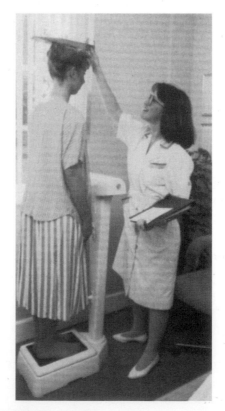

FIGURE NUMBER: 13.21 – Measuring weight and height.

Weight measurement

Method:

■ Instruct the client to wear minimum clothing (record this to ensure that the same clothing is worn each time the weight is taken), with bare feet. Ask the client to stand still in the centre of the weighing machine and to look directly ahead.

■ Read the weight, record it on the client's card and inform the client.

Body measurement

Measurements to be recorded:

■ Bust/chest
■ Waist
■ Hips
■ Upper thigh
■ Lower thigh
■ Upper arms

Method:

■ Select a tape measure that is in good condition, not frayed or stretched. Always ensure that the tape is level on the body part and not twisted. Do not pull the tape measure. Use the nearest prominent bony point as a marker. This will ensure that the tape will be placed at the same level each time. Thin elastic can be used to indicate the level.

■ Instruct the client to remove all clothing except pants (very self-conscious women may keep a bra on, but they should wear the same bra each time the measurements are taken), stand in bare feet and maintain a good posture, with the arms to the side.

Bust or chest

■ Bring the tape around the back, under the armpit and around the nipple line.
■ Record the measurement and inform the client.

Waist

■ Give a circle of narrow elastic to the client and ask her to place this at the narrowest part, i.e. her natural waistline. Measure just above the elastic. For males, measure at the level of the navel.
■ Record the measurement and inform the client.

Hips

■ Place the tape around the widest part of the hips and measure. Then measure the distance of the tape from the greater trochanter: this will ensure that the tape is placed at the same level next time.
■ Record the measurement and inform the client.

Right and left upper thigh

- Again, use a circle of narrow elastic. Place this around the widest part of the thigh. Measure the distance from the elastic to the top of the patella.
- Place the tape around the leg just above the elastic.
- Record the measurement and inform the client.

Right and left lower thigh

- Use a circle of narrow elastic and place it two to three inches above the top of the patella.
- Place the tape around the leg just above the elastic.
- Record the measurement and inform the client.

Right and left upper arms

- Place a circle of narrow elastic around the widest part of the upper arm. Measure the distance from this to the olecranon process.
- Place the tape around the arm just above the elastic.
- Record the measurement and inform the client.

Midriff

- For women whose objective is to lose body weight, measurement of the midriff is necessary. Measure around the midriff two to three inches below the xiphoid process.

Calf

- For those wishing to build up the calf muscle, measure around the wide part of the calf and note the distance from the tape to the lateral malleolus. Use the same distance next time.

Testing for muscle strength

Muscle strength is measured by how much weight the muscle is able to move. This is tested using weights or a grip test or by pulling against machines.

Weight lift

- Select a suitable stable starting position.
- Select an appropriate weight and check that it is secure.
- Isolate the movement to the muscle being tested.
- Ask the client to lift the weight smoothly to the full inner range three times. If an extra lift is possible, the weight must be increased.
- Ask the client to rest for one to two minutes and repeat the lift with extra weight. The weight that is lifted smoothly two or three times indicates the strength.
- Record the weight.

Grip test

- Make sure the client is holding the grip comfortably in the hand. In the standing position the client lifts the arm above the head, lowers the arm and squeezes as hard as possible. Repeat three times.
- Record the highest reading.

There are a variety of machines on the market designed for testing strength. Read the manufacturer's instructions very carefully, and test a colleague to ensure that you fully understand the procedure.

Exercises such as push-ups and sit-ups are sometimes used to give an indication of fitness, but these are not measurable.

Muscle tone

It is possible to obtain some indication of muscle strength by applying manual resistance to muscle action and feeling the degree of tone within the muscle. This will only provide a rough guide, as it is not possible to quantify the strength but only to categorise it into poor, moderate, good, very good or excellent. Muscles that are easily tested in this way are the biceps and triceps, the abdominals, gluteus maximus and the hip abductors and adductors.

Method:
- Position the client in crook lying. This position can be maintained throughout and avoids moving the client unnecessarily.
- One hand must be placed over the working muscle to feel the tone, while the other hand is used to resist the movement.

Biceps strength

- The client bends the elbow to the mid-point of the range.
- Place one hand over the biceps on the anterior aspect of the upper arm. Grasp the wrist with the other.
- Instruct the client to bend the elbow while you stop the movement. Feel the increased tone with the hand placed over the muscle. Is the strength you are feeling poor, moderate, good, very good or excellent? This value judgement becomes easier with practice.
- Record the result.

Triceps strength

- With one hand, cover the triceps on the posterior aspect of the upper arm. Keep the other hand around the wrist.
- Instruct the client to straighten the elbow against resistance. Feel the increased tone with the hand placed over the muscle, and assess the strength.
- Record the result.

Abdominal strength (particularly rectus abdominus)

- Place one hand over the abdominals.
- Instruct the client to perform a curl-up (lifting head and shoulders with chin on chest). If this is done with ease, the free hand can be placed over the sternum and resistance given to the curl-up.
- Feel the increased tone with the hand placed on the abdominals, and assess the strength.
- Record the result.

Gluteus maximus strength

- Instruct the client to lift his or her bottom up off the bed and tighten the buttocks. (A sandbag weight can be placed over the pelvis to provide resistance.)
- Place a hand over the gluteus maximus.
- Feel the increased tone and judge the strength.
- Record the result.

Abductor strength

- Straighten the client's leg.
- Place one hand over the abductors on the outer aspect of the thigh above the greater trochanter.
- Place the other hand under the ankle to cup it.
- Instruct the client to 'push out' towards you. Resist the movement, using the hand at the ankle to push inwards.
- Feel the increased tone in the abductors and judge the strength.
- Record the result.

Adductor strength

- Keep the client's leg straight and pulled outwards.
- Keep the hand under the ankle.
- Place the other hand over the adductors on the inner aspect of the thigh (upper third).
- Instruct the client to pull the leg inwards towards the other leg. Resist the movement, using the hand at the ankle to pull outwards.
- Feel the increased tone in the adductors and judge the strength.
- Record the result.

Cardio-respiratory endurance

This may be tested using a treadmill or bicycle ergometer. If this specialised equipment is not available, the step test can be used.

Three-minute step test

Equipment:
- Twelve-inch step

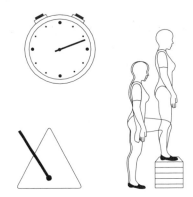

FIGURE NUMBER: 13.22 – Step test.

- Metronome
- Timing clock/stopwatch
- Stethoscope for measuring heart rate (or take the pulse with the index and middle fingers over the radial artery).

Method:
- Explain the test to the client, demonstrating how to step up and down for three minutes at 24 steps per minute.
- Ask the client to practise.
- Set the metronome to 96 clicks per minute. With each click a foot must move, i.e. click 1: right foot onto step; click 2: left foot onto step; click 3: right foot down off step; click 4: left foot down off step.
- Time the client for three minutes.

Then sit and quickly take the client's pulse or heart rate for one minute. (Count for 30 seconds and multiply by two.) The pulse rate is an excellent indication of cardio-vascular efficiency. If the recorded heart rate is above the maximum heart rate recommended for that client, the client is unfit and must exercise with caution. The client should exercise at a target rate below 50 per cent of MHR. If there is any sign of stress, stop exercising and seek medical advice. As fitness increases and cardio-vascular efficiency increases, the heart rate will decrease and target rate will increase to 60 percent. As a rough guide, compare the test result with Table 13.1.

Maximum heart rate (MHR)

To calculate Maximum Heart Rate use 220 minus the age of client. Healthy individuals should exercise at a target or training rate of 60–85 per cent of their maximal heart rate. Those at the fair to poor end of the above table would exercise at 60 per cent of the MHR. The fit individuals at the excellent end of the table would need to exercise at the higher end (80–85 per cent) to achieve sufficient overload.

Table 13.1
The range of heart rates after three minutes' stepping

	Men aged 20–46	Women aged 20–46
Excellent	81–90	79–84
Good	99–102	90–97
Above average	103–112	106–109
Average	120–121	118–119
Below average	123–125	122–124
Fair	127–130	129–134
Poor	136–138	137–145

(Adapted from YMCA Y's Way to Fitness.)

Body composition

Equipment:

■ Skin-fold callipers.

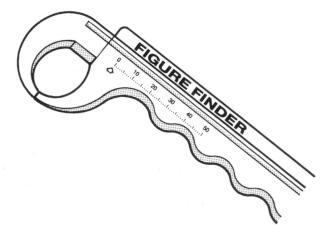

FIGURE NUMBER: 13.23 – Skin fold callipers.

Method:
■ Identify the locations of the skin folds (see Table 13.2).
■ Hold the callipers in the dominant hand.
■ Pinch the skin fold with the thumb and forefinger of the other hand.
■ Hold the callipers perpendicular to the skin fold and place the pads very near the thumb and forefinger.
■ Close or release the callipers, depending on type.

Table 13.2
The locations of the skin folds

Women	Men
Supra-iliac fold diagonally above the crest of the ilium	Abdominal fold vertically 2 cm lateral to umbilicus
Anterior thigh fold vertically midway between knee and hip	Anterior thigh fold vertically midway between knee and hip
Triceps fold vertically midway between elbow and shoulder	Chest fold diagonally halfway between nipple and crease of axilla

Table 13.3
The range of body fat percentages

Women	Men	Rating
less than 25 mm	less than 22 mm	excellent
25 mm–42 mm	22 mm–34 mm	good
43 mm–65 mm	35 mm–73 mm	average
66 mm–82 mm	74 mm–90 mm	fair
over 82 mm	over 90 mm	poor

- Record the measurement.
- Take three or more readings at each skin fold to gain consistency.

The consistent readings at each site are then added together, averaged, and compared with the Table 13.3. This will indicate whether or not there is a need to reduce weight. Measurements may be taken every four to six weeks and compared with previous readings to indicate weight gain or loss. The importance of body composition is explained in full in chapter 9.

Lung capacity measurement

Equipment:
- Spirometer and accessories.

Method:
- Ask the client to stand straight, and clip on the nose clip.
- Instruct the client to fill the lungs completely with air with a single deep inhalation, then place the mouth around the disinfected mouthpiece and ensure a perfect seal.

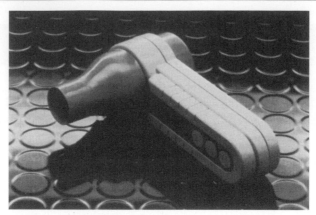

FIGURE NUMBER: 13.24 – Hand held spirometer.

- The client should then breathe out as hard as possible for as long as possible.
- Take three attempts to ensure accurate reading, pausing for three to four minutes between each attempt.
- Read and record the measurements and compare them with charts for normal ranges.

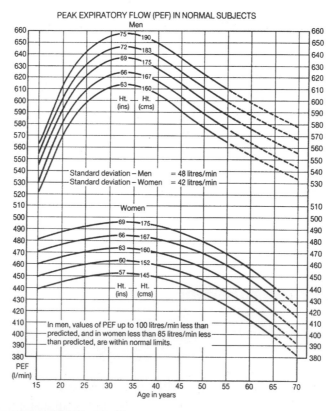

FIGURE NUMBER: 13.25 – Lung capacities of men and women.

Blood pressure

Equipment:

■ A sphygmomanometer is used to measure blood pressure. The modern models usually found in fitness centres are automatic and give a digital readout. These differ from the models used medically, where a stethoscope is used over the radial artery at the elbow, the sounds during systole and diastole are listened to and the corresponding pressure level for each is read.

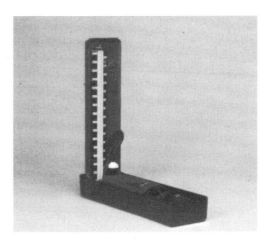

FIGURE NUMBER: 13.26 – A sphygmomanometer.

Method:

■ Normal blood pressure for a young resting adult is about $\frac{120\ \text{(systolic)}}{80\ \text{(diastolic)}}$ mm Hg but this varies considerably with activity, emotion and age. Blood pressure tends to rise as we get older. Systolic pressure in adults at rest averages 110–150 mm Hg, diastolic 60–65 mm Hg. *Anyone giving repeated systolic pressure readings of more than of 140 mm Hg should consult a doctor for a check-up before exercising.*

Flexibility

It is possible to measure lower back and hamstring flexibility for the fit client.

Equipment:

■ A box or stool with a tape attached

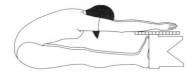

FIGURE NUMBER: 13.27 – Flexibility test. (Seat and reach.)

Method:

- The client should sit with legs stretched out and feet against the box or stool, and with arms stretched forward.
- Ask the client to breathe out, reach forward and slide the hands along the stool. Read the distance at the middle finger. If the box has a slider, the client should push this forward with the hands and the reading is taken.
- Measure for three attempts and record the best result.

TASK

Work with a partner. Practise the different assessment on each other.

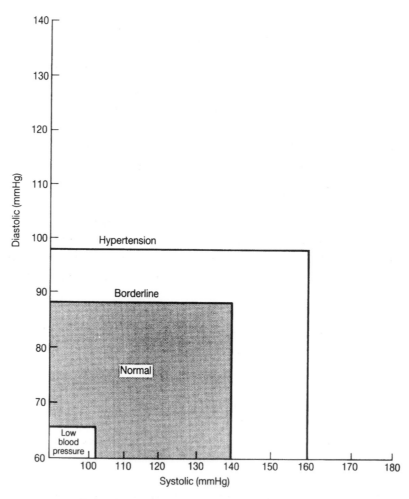

FIGURE NUMBER: 13.28 – Blood pressure range.

Chapter 14
Exercise classes

Exercise classes provide many different forms of exercise, for example general keep fit, aerobic, dance, step, weight loss, line dancing, relaxation, etc. Although they differ in the type of exercise offered, certain basic principles apply to all.

It is desirable, though not always possible, to organise classes so that there is parity within the groups, for example similar fitness levels, similar age groups and similar desired outcomes. It is very important to recognise and allow for individual differences within a group: different intellectual levels, fitness levels, body shapes, health, previous experience, lifestyles, age and motivation.

Each class member must be instructed to work at his or her own pace, and heart rate must be used to monitor intensity. No-one should exceed their maximum heart rate – see page 146.

Remember: beginners must work at 60 per cent of the maximum heart rate and increase to 80 per cent as fitness develops. All members must practice taking the radial pulse for fifteen seconds and multiplying by four. They must continue to monitor the pulse at intervals throughout the class. Members must stop exercising if the target heart rate is exceeded or if there are any signs of stress.

LEARN
To work out a client's maximum heart rate (MHR) subtract their age from 220. Heart rate must stay below this when exercising. The target rate will be 60–90 percent of this.

LEARNING NEW SKILLS

The theories of learning apply to both individual and class teaching. Members attend in order to acquire new skills, which will aid the achievement of set goals or objectives. These goals will vary from person to person. In order to help the members of a class to achieve these goals, the teacher must organise the lessons so that optimum learning and performance can take place.

The teaching of a skill requires demonstration (by the teacher) followed by practice by the members, but before this can occur it is essential to prepare adequately the environment where the learning is to take place.

As previously outlined, the environment must be warm, well ventilated, free from distractions and external noise and safe. The floor must be firm, smooth and, preferably, sprung. All equipment must be checked and organised before the commencement of the class so that the sequence of the lesson is not broken, as interruption of any kind interferes with the learning process. Members must be acknowledged and greeted in a friendly and reassuring way. This ensures that members feel physically and psychologically 'safe'.

Learning a new exercise is a very complex process. It is useful to consider the nature of a skill and how it may be defined.

- Curzon (1976) defines a skill as 'a series of learned acts requiring simultaneous or sequential co-ordination'.
- The UK Department of Employment (Curzon, 1976) defines a skill as 'an organised and co-ordinated pattern of mental and physical activity'.

The essential features of a skilled performance are:

- accuracy of timing;
- anticipation of movement;
- economy of effort;
- grace and precision of movement;
- the overall flow of the movement.

To enable members of the class to attain this level, the teacher must analyse each skill and break it down into a sequence of separate movements, which are then joined together to make the whole performance. The acquisition of a skill requires the use of both receptor and effector processes, in other words effective co-ordination of mind and muscle. There are many theories on the learning of motor skills.

One theory suggests that the learner must pass through three overlapping stages: (Fitts and Posner, 1967)

Stage 1

- The *cognitive phase* – this involves knowledge of the skill and understanding of what is required. The learner analyses the task and tries to understand what is to be done and how to do it. He or she knows when errors are made but is unsure how to correct them. At this stage co-ordination is poor, concentration levels high, cues and correction must be given frequently and common errors pointed out. At this stage the skill can be broken down into simple parts to make learning easier.

Stage 2
■ The *associative or motor phase* – as a result of practice, errors are gradually eliminated. Correct patterns are established and, although errors are still made, they are corrected with minimal prompting. Movement is more consistent and effective, the learner can consider finer detail and can link sequences together to produce skilled performance. The learner can now recognise and correct his/her mistakes. Few cues are given at this stage as too much feedback makes the learner too dependent.

Stage 3
■ The *autonomous phase* – skills are performed automatically and require little thought. Errors have been eliminated, speed and accuracy increased and the effects of stress reduced. The motor skill is now highly developed.

Feedback

It is the instructor's role to guide members of the class through these stages and to provide continuous feedback throughout. They must be informed of their current progress and told how to improve it. Millar distinguishes between two forms of feedback:
■ *Action feedback*, which provides knowledge of current progress. Actions are corrected as they are performed. The instructor must therefore provide spoken cues during the performance of the exercise, such as 'eyes front', 'hold the head up', 'shoulders down', 'knees higher', 'do not stretch too far', 'do not lift too high', 'curl back slowly from below', etc.
■ *Learning feedback*, which provides information that enables the student to improve next time. This might include cues such as 'that was a good attempt, but some people did not keep the back straight', 'well done, but keep those tummies in', 'well done, but watch that you roll the pelvis backwards before you come up' or 'I obviously didn't explain that exercise clearly', followed by further explanation and demonstration. In this way, members can correct their performance and will move quickly into the autonomous phase.

Feedback must therefore be given as each exercise or part of an exercise is being performed, and also at the end. This enables the learner to discriminate between correct and incorrect patterns at an early stage and thus avoids incorrect patterns being reinforced.

Many corrective statements and cues will be required for new members of a class or when members are learning a new exercise, but as the skill is mastered fewer cues are needed. Positive value statements such as 'good', 'that's better', 'well done' or 'great' will encourage members and increase motivation. It is important always to encourage and never to put anyone down, nor draw attention to poor performance or embarrass the learner. If only one or two members are not performing correctly, give a general corrective statement, or catch their eye and say 'watch me', or explain the correction quietly and privately at the end of the class.

Feedback is essential as it provides knowledge of correct or incorrect performance, reinforces the correct response and increases motivation.

MOTIVATION

Motivation may be defined as the drive within an individual to take an appropriate course of action in order to satisfy a need.

Motivation heightens performance. The good instructor, teacher or coach is able to stimulate the student's own motivation. The instructor can ensure that the class is well organised and administered and that the teaching style is enthusiastic, positive, concerned, caring, knowledgeable and safe. A high level of expertise must be demonstrated at all times, both in theoretical knowledge and in practical demonstration.

Motivation is greatly enhanced by encouraging and promoting feelings of satisfaction, achievement, recognition, responsibility, advancement, personal growth and success, enjoyment and fun.

However, poor, unpleasant surroundings, lack of organisation and safety, feelings of dissatisfaction, failure and embarrassment, lack of interest and unrealistic goals that are not achievable are all demotivators and must be avoided.

Setting objectives or goals

This is a very important part of planning for group or individual exercises. The members' aspirations and the possibilities of realising them must be fully discussed. When members are involved in setting the objectives they know where they are going and can better help themselves to get there, so motivation is increased. The objective may be to:

- increase cardio-respiratory fitness;
- improve muscle strength;
- improve flexibility;
- reduce fatty deposits;
- improve body shape;
- improve posture;
- correct figure faults;
- improve speed and skill.

Objectives must be realistic and they must be achievable within a limited time scale. A rounded five foot tall endomorph will never be tall and slender – that goal would be unrealistic – but to lose fat and improve body shape would be achievable and realistic. The setting of long-term goals and short-term goals, which are continually monitored through regular assessment, will increase motivation. Once the objectives have been agreed, planning the strategy can begin. Consider the age and ability of participants. Organise groups into beginners, intermediate or advanced. Lesson plans for each session should be prepared: these are necessary as a record of work and show progression. Consider the type of exercises required to meet objectives. Consider intensity, frequency and duration.

Each lesson plan should include:
- the objectives;
- the sequence of activities;
- the time allowed for each part of the sequence;
- the music, if used;
- the equipment necessary;
- any comments or notes.

An example can be found in Table 14.1

Objective:
- To correct lordosis and improve muscle balance
- To reduce weight.

THE ORGANISATION OF A CLASS

- Prepare the room before the members arrive.
- Ensure that the lighting and ventilation are adequate.
- Check that the floor is firm, clean and smooth.
- If mats are to be used, make sure there is one for each person.
- Locate the first-aid box and note all the exits.
- Check that the area is clear of equipment or apparatus or anything that may be a safety hazard.
- Select all required equipment or apparatus.
- Check that the equipment and apparatus is in sound working order and safe to use. Ensure that there is enough to go round.
- Arrange all the equipment neatly at one end of the room well away from the working area.
- Select the music tapes or records and stack them in order of use.
- Check that the music centre or player is working.
- Provide a large clock with a second hand to be used when monitoring maximum heart rate.
- Shower and change into appropriate clothes. Remember that you set the standard for the class. Wear clean, unrestricting, absorbent, smart clothing and suitable footwear (see chapter 13).
- Tie the hair back and remove jewellery.

When the members arrive:
- Greet the members warmly, using their names where possible; at the very least, make eye contact or wave to show each member that they are recognised.

Table 14.1
Sample lesson plan

Activity	Time	Equipment	Music	Comments
Discussion of previous week's class including any problems, and outline today's exercises	5–10 minutes	–	– –	explain that these objectives require different exercises: ■ to reduce weight – aerobics; ■ to correct lordosis – strengthening abdominals and stretching back extensors
Warm-up: alternate heel raising, walking on the spot and around the room, marching with knees high, pelvic tilt, circle pelvis, twist trunk, shoulder circling, arm circling, chest press	10 minutes	–	any suitable music for age group or time of year	begin slowly and increase pace. Work on large muscle groups. Include exercises for mobilising and pulse raising.
Stretch: erector spinae, hip flexors (select from chapter 11)	5 minutes	rolled towel	–	slow gentle static stretch, hold for a count of ten, repeat
Aerobic section	15 minutes	step	theme music, faster tempo	work to target heart rate. Take pulse every five minutes, stop if above target, work harder if too low (see chapter 7)
Strengthening exercises	10 minutes	medicine ball, sand bag	–	use crook lying curl-ups for the abdominal muscles and leg extension for the gluteus maximus and hamstrings. Caution: do not extend the lower back, keep the hips on the floor
Cool-down: select from chapter 12	10 minutes	–	any music with a slow tempo	keep moving – do not stand still
Stretch				
Discussion: feedback to and from class participants	5 minutes or longer if time allows	–	–	Allow the clients time to ask questions and clarify uncertainties. Give them positive feedback. Leave on a 'high' note.

- Make a point of greeting and speaking to new members and introduce them to other members.
- Point out toilets, exits, first-aid box, safety procedures.
- Register all participants.
- Carry out a consultation or assessment of each new member and ensure that he or she has read the instructions (see chapter 13) and signed the consent form.
- Check that members are wearing suitable unrestricting clothing and suitable footwear.
- Check that hair is tied back and jewellery is removed.
- Begin the class on time.

During the class:
- Step confidently in front of the class, speak clearly and make sure that those at the back can hear. Use the voice to good effect: change the tone to govern speed, rhythm, intensity and effort.
- Remember that you are the role model for the class. Therefore, develop a warm, friendly, enthusiastic, positive approach. Good posture and an alert and efficient manner will set the tone of the class. Do not fidget or develop irritating mannerisms such as tossing the hair or rubbing the leg.
- When demonstrating an exercise, ensure that your performance is as accurate and perfect as possible. Poor demonstration means poor performance and ineffective exercise, which may also impose stresses on the body, causing strain and injury.
- Become an educator. Outline the objectives. Explain the reasons for and the effects of each exercise. Explain the health benefits of exercise (see chapter 12).
- Take time to explain and teach new exercises.
- Stress that each individual must work at his or her own pace and target heart rate. He or she must not exceed the maximum heart rate. New members should work at 60 per cent of MHR working up to 80–85 per cent (see chapter 13). Make sure that each member can calculate this and know how to take their pulse.
- Following the demonstration, give clear, simple commands and corrective cues, particularly in the early stages.
- Break complicated exercises down into manageable 'chunks'. Teach one part at a time until each is well executed and then perform them together as a whole.
- Give encouragement to enhance motivation, i.e. 'well done', 'that's good', 'much better', 'that's great', 'a great effort', etc.
- Watch for signs of stress.
- Tell the client to stop exercising if there are signs of stress such as profuse sweating, breathlessness, tightness in the chest, pain in the chest or arms, pain in the back or any joints, faintness or dizziness, headache, nausea or a heart rate above the maximum.
- Members must not be made to feel that they are in competition with others, nor under pressure to keep up with the instructor. If possible, organise classes into easy (beginners), intermediate and advanced to accommodate fitness levels, or organise them into age groups, in order to maintain some parity within the groups. Allow time for discussion before the session commences. This may cover any problems experienced during or after the previous class, any minor injuries or joint problems experienced or

any interesting new information for discussion. Explain the importance of maintaining good posture and give advice on protecting the back, neck and knees.

■ Explain the importance of breathing normally and not holding the breath. Instruct members to breathe in before an effort or on release and to breathe out on the effort.

■ Give reasons for the importance of the warm-up (see chapter 12). Emphasise that even if members turn up late they must not join the class until they have completed the ten-minute warm-up. They must do this at the edge or back of the class and then join in the other exercises. Explain the importance of stretching and the associated hazards (see chapter 9).

■ Explain the importance of the cool-down in allowing the body to return slowly to the balanced state. Explain why cool-down exercises should be performed while continuously moving around or end with lying down for rest and breathing.

■ Allow time at the end for participants to ask questions and clarify any uncertain points.

■ Give feedback regarding the session

■ Outline the activities for the next and future sessions – remind them of goals.

■ Clear away all equipment and leave the room in a clean and tidy state.

AEROBIC CLASS

The American College of Sports Medicine defines aerobic activity as follows:

'Aerobic activity is that requiring continuous, rhythmic use of large muscle groups at 60–90 per cent of the maximum heart rate and 50–85 per cent of maximum oxygen uptake for 20–60 minutes at least three times per week.'

The main effects of aerobic exercises are:
■ an increase in cardio-respiratory fitness;
■ a reduction of fatty deposits, with resultant weight loss;
■ an increase in muscular endurance;
■ the maintenance of bone mass.

Types of aerobic class

There are various activities designed to keep the body in continuous rhythmic motion and the list is continually growing. We now have high, moderate and low impact aerobics, step, dance and water aerobics.

High-impact aerobics, where both feet leave the ground, are no longer recommended as they place members at risk of injury due to continuous jarring.

Low impact, where one foot always stays in contact with the ground and the knees are slightly bent, are safer. Moderate impact will include some high impact, but consists mainly of low-impact work. It is more desirable to concentrate on duration and intensity than on impact.

Duration is increased by performing more repetitions. Intensity is increased by using longer and higher steps: from jogging to marching to high stepping. The arm position can change from waist level or at the sides to shoulder level and above the head. Light ankle and wrist weights can be used. Fitter members can exaggerate their movements, taking bigger steps and travelling more.

Energy expenditure will depend on the intensity and duration of the exercises. Low intensity long duration movements will utilise the aerobic energy system, this means glycogen and fat. The higher, faster and longer the movements, the greater will be the energy expenditure. However if the exercises are too intense and fast the anaerobic system will switch in. This will use only glycogen and result in an accumulation of lactic acid.

As with all classes, it is important to begin gradually. This allows the body to adapt to increased demand. Exercises should begin with low-intensity work, build up to peak intensity and decrease gradually.

- The heart must adapt to maintain adequate blood supply to the working muscles.
- Blood flow will be diverted from the organs to the muscles.
- The respiratory rate must increase gradually to ensure adequate ventilation. A too-rapid increase in breathing will result in hyper-ventilation and side cramps.

Plan the class as outlined on page 309. Always include a warm-up, stretching, main core exercises and a cool-down. Relaxation and breathing exercises may also be included if appropriate.

> **LEARN**
> Instruct members to go from standing to lying by going down on the hands and knees, rolling onto their side and then onto the back, with the reverse procedure for standing up again.)

Selecting music

Selecting music is an important part of the planning. The music will set the 'mood' of the class, it provides timing for the exercises and it keeps the class working together. It helps to provide interest, fun and enjoyment, and also increases motivation. When selecting music, consider the age range and lifestyle of the clients where possible; for example, younger clients will enjoy contemporary pop music, while older clients may prefer 1960s music, big bands, folk, country and western, gospel or square dance music. Consider also the time of year, for example Christmas music or summer songs. If the class is mixed, use a variety of music, with something to suit everyone. Ask class members if they have favourite records or tapes that they would like to use.

Planning exercises to music

The choreography, that is the planning of the movements and sequences of music, must be done well in advance. This is difficult at first, but becomes easier with practice. Watch exercise videos, noting how the steps match the beat of the music. Watch modern dance and ballet, observing how foot, trunk and arm movements fit the music.

List all the foot and leg movements that you may wish to include in the class. Then list all the arm movements that may be performed on their own or to accompany the leg movements. For examples, see Table 14.2.

Table 14.2
Sample lesson plan

Leg movement	Arm movement
Heel raise	Hands on waist (wing)
Jog	Hands on shoulders (bend)
March	Arms out to side or front
High knee march	Arms on head
Walk	Arms reach up (shoulder press)
Steps forward, back, to side	Alternate arms reach up
Step touches	Alternate arms reach sideways or forwards (chest press)
Step and kick	Swinging forward and back
Step and knee lift	Sideways clap
Step, knee lift and kick	Shoulder shrugging
Plié (caution)	Shoulder circling
Grapevine (cross one leg in front of or behind the other)	Air punching forwards and upwards
Hopscotch	Across body swing
Rabbit hops	

In the same way list floor and stretch exercises.

Select music to suit the class. Listen carefully to each piece of music and note:
- the rhythm – this is the regular pattern of sound which will dictate the style of the exercise routine;
- the beat – these are the pulsations of music. The beat is very important as a step or movement will accompany each beat;
- the timing or number of beats in each bar. Music with two or four beats in the bar is best for class work. Waltz time (three beats in a bar) can be used for stretching;

■ the tempo – the rate at which the music is played. The American book *Aerobics Dance-Exercise* suggests that slow tempos of 100–120 beats per minute are suitable for warm-up and cool-down, and under 100 beats per minute for stretch and floor exercises, while faster tempos of 130–160 should be used for aerobics and dance.

Having listened to the music, select from the list of exercises suitable movements and patterns to fit the music. Practise these thoroughly yourself and record each movement and series of movements. Movements or patterns are usually repeated four to six times. Plan movements for the warm-up, stretch, main core – building up the intensity and then easing down again – and cool-down. Note cues for good posture, breathing and accurate movements.

TASK 1

Work with a partner.
■ Prepare a first lesson plan for a 30-year-old client who wants to lose weight and improve the strength of the abdominals.
■ Explain the reasons for your choice of exercises to the client.

TASK 2

Work with a partner.
■ Prepare a working area for an aerobics class.
■ Instruct a client on how to lie down on the floor and come up again.
■ Teach a client correct breathing, using the diaphragm and lower ribs.

TASK 3

■ Plan an aerobics lesson for a group of 30–45-year-olds who are moderately fit.
■ Discuss the reasoning behind your selection of exercises.

TASK 4

Work in a group.
■ Teach any six exercises to the group without music.

TASK 5

Work in a group.

- Select a piece of suitable music and plan a sequence of movements to fit the music which may be used in an aerobics class.
- Teach these exercises to a small group.

Remember to:

- listen to the music first;
- demonstrate the movement correctly;
- break the movement down into parts;
- teach each part thoroughly, with and without music,
- link all the parts together;
- practise the entire sequence.

Chapter 15
First Aid for sports injuries

Attempting to diagnose or treat any injury without specialist medical training is dangerous practice. The rate and success of recovery will depend on accurate diagnosis, followed by careful rehabilitation. Inappropriate treatment can cause further damage and permanently impair function. However, knowing what action to take immediately before medical attention is available can reduce the extent of tissue damage. The trainer is often the first person on the scene following injury and must make rapid and crucial decisions based on knowledge and experience. Everyone connected with sport should be familiar with the principles of first aid, as immediate action may be needed.

Prevention of injury

Every precaution should be taken to prevent the occurrence of injury. Factors which contribute to injuries are:

- Inadequate or inappropriate training: plan well-designed exercise schemes showing gradual progression, give accurate instruction.
- Inadequate warm-up and cool-down.
- Faulty equipment and poor surfaces: select a suitable venue with appropriate facilities and good surfaces, check equipment.
- Improper use of equipment.
- Inappropriate footwear or clothing.
- Unsuitable weather conditions.
- Incomplete recovery following a previous injury: ensure adequate rest, relaxation and recovery time.
- Activities inappropriate to age and fitness levels: ensure appropriate fitness assessment prior to undertaking sport or exercise and also on return after injury.

- Intensive competition, resulting in risk taking.
- Dehydration and poor nutrition.
- Exercising when there are contra-indications.
- Poor exercise technique: maintain good body alignment throughout, practise correct technique and breathing patterns.

Immediate assessment of injury

It is vitally important to assess the situation as soon as injury occurs. The injured person should not be moved until a preliminary examination has been carried out.

Breathing

Watch for chest movement or check nose and mouth for air flow. If there is no rise and fall of the chest, and you feel no movement of air, begin mouth to mouth resuscitation.

Heartbeat

Feel for pulse: radial pulse at wrist, carotid pulse at throat behind wind pipe. If there is no pulse, begin cardiac compression.

Broken bones

If for any reason fractures are suspected, do not move the casualty more than is absolutely necessary. This is particularly important if there is damage to the spine. Moving a casualty with damage to their spine can result in permanent paralysis.

Bleeding

Any profuse bleeding should be stemmed by applying firm even pressure directly over the area, preferably over a sterile dressing. Protect yourself from blood contamination.

Other injuries

Look for wounds, cuts, abrasions, signs of joint damage, e.g., pain, ligament sprains, muscle and tendon strain and tears.

Immediate treatment

The quicker the treatment is administered following injury the greater the chance of speedy full recovery. Treatment should start immediately where possible and certainly within 24 hours.

Treatment is generally aimed to:
- preserve life;
- promote healing;
- return body to normal function.

More specific aims are:
- to prevent further damage;

- to reduce the inflammatory response;
- to reduce pain, swelling and stiffness;
- to gradually stretch, mobilise and strengthen the affected tissues;
- to maintain full strength and condition of unaffected body parts.

Fast action limits damage: for immediate action, think 'RICED':
- **R** – rest and immobilisation to prevent further damage;
- **I** – apply ice immediately for vasoconstriction and to prevent secondary damage;
- **C** – compression to the area to reduce swelling;
- **E** – elevation (using gravity to assist drainage from the area);
- **D** – diagnosis by a doctor either on site, in a surgery or in hospital.

Rest

Further damage to an injured part can be prevented by resting and immobilising the part. The casualty should be moved only if absolutely necessary, to facilitate breathing, to remove from the field of play or to prevent further injury. The injured part should be rested and supported correctly using splints, tubular, stocking or crepe bandages as necessary. These give firmer support if a layer of cotton wool is wrapped around the area before applying the bandage. If leg fractures are suspected, the good leg can be used as a splint by tying the two legs together, or long strips of wood can be used and bound to the leg until medical treatment is available. A stretcher will then be needed to transport the casualty.

The casualty should rest for 24–48 hours after injury and should not put weight on an injured leg. Elbow or axillary crutches should be used, or support can be given by a person on either side with the casualty hopping on the good leg.

If the arm is seriously injured, a sling should be used for support. A triangular sling is placed around the lower arm and supporting the elbow. The long end is taken over the opposite shoulder and the short end over the injured side, the two ends are tied at the back of the neck. If the injury is below the elbow, the forearm should be supported upwards to assist drainage.

Crutch walking

Measure the crutches carefully. There should be a space the width of three fingers (i.e. 6 cm) between the top of the crutch and the axilla (arm pit), otherwise pressure will damage the nerves in the region. The hand rest should be level with the crease of the wrist or the styloid process.

Two point walking should be used when both crutches are moved forward together: the casualty pushes on the hand rest, straighten the elbows and hops to the crutches – do not hop *through* the crutches as this can result in loss of balance and falling backwards. Do not place the crutches too far forward as they will slip. The rhythm will be:
- lift and move crutches forward;
- push on hands;
- straighten elbows;
- hop to the crutches.

For going upstairs, put foot first, then crutches; for coming downstairs, put crutches first, then foot. Elbow crutches are used in a similar way, but do not give as much support.

Ice

Ice should be placed over the injured area as soon as possible. This will reduce the metabolic rate and oxygen requirement of the cells around the periphery of the injury. These cells would not receive oxygen because of the damage to blood vessels and would die resulting in secondary injury. Cold will also reduce internal bleeding and swelling as the blood vessels constrict, reducing fluid exudate and bruising.

Care must be taken when applying ice to the area, as there is a risk of producing ice burns if the ice comes into contact with the skin over a prolonged period. The area should be covered with oil for ice cube massage, or a tea towel should be used between the skin and the ice when using ice packs.

There are various ways of applying ice:
1 Stroke the oiled skin with an ice cube, keeping the ice moving over the area slowly.
2 Ice cubes can be shattered and placed in a towel, which is wrapped around the injury over a tea towel.
3 Freezer packs or even frozen food such as a packet of peas can be used; place them over a tea towel covering the area, and hold in place by another towel. These packs are very useful as they can be refrozen and reused.
4 Ankle and wrist injuries can be immersed in iced water in a bucket or bowl. The part is held in the water for as long as is tolerable, is removed for a new minutes and then re-immersed.

Ice should be applied for at least 10–15 minutes, increasing to 30 minutes, unless the skin is sensitive and the area feels uncomfortable. The skin should turn colour: pink for pale skin but darker for dark skin.

Ice should be applied every two to three hours, initially working down to three times a day as healing progresses and the swelling subsides.

Note: Heat should never be used in the acute stage of injury as it increases metabolic rate, and produces vasodilation, which increases blood flow and swelling. Heat may be used after healing has taken place (usually in 6–12 days), but only after the bruising turns yellow.

Compression

This means applying pressure to the area, which helps to limit the bleeding into the tissues. An elasticated tubular or crepe bandage may be used. Additional pressure can be applied if a layer of cotton wool is applied to the area before bandaging. Do not use non-elasticated bandages on a recent injury; the strapping needs some stretch to allow for swelling.

The strapping must not be too tight, as it will restrict the circulation. If the swelling increases, the pressure under the strapping will increase, and this will produce further restriction and damage. Check the swelling and the colour of the skin and nails beyond the strapping; white/grey skin and blue nails indicate that the strapping is too tight, in which case the bandage should be released.

Elevation

The injured part should be supported in elevation whenever possible. Gravity will then assist the drainage of any fluid exudate away from the area. This will help to reduce the pressure within the tissues and the pain around the damaged area.

Diagnosis

Accurate diagnosis is crucial for maximum recovery. Seek medical advice as quickly as possible if there is doubt about the injury, and for any of the following conditions:

- Head injuries
- Headache, nausea, vomiting or dizziness following head injuries
- Pains in the neck or symptoms down the arms such as tingling or numbness
- Pains in the back and down the legs, or numbness
- Breathing difficulties or pains in the chest
- Fracture or suspected fracture
- Dislocation of a joint, or severe injury to a joint or ligament
- Profuse bleeding and deep or large wounds
- Severe muscle and tendon injuries
- Abdominal or groin pain
- Eye injuries

Summary of precautions

- Do not move a casualty with injuries to the spine.
- Do not move a casualty with fractured bones, more than is absolutely necessary.
- Apply bandages and strapping firmly, but not too tightly as too much pressure may restrict the circulation.
- Check the limbs beyond the strapping for cold, white or blue colouration which indicates lack of circulation – loosen the strap immediately if this is the case.
- Do not apply heat in any form to the injured area, i.e. do not use heat lamps, hot packs, hot baths, showers, ultra-sound, diathermy, hot towels or any liniments.
- Do not massage the injured area.
- Do not exercise through the pain or use electrical stimulation.
- Do not allow the injured person to drink alcohol.

Types of injury

Injuries can be divided into two categories:

1 *Acute injuries:* Traumatic injuries which happen suddenly due to some external force or internal stress; these produce sudden pain, swelling, bruising or wounds.
2 *Chronic injuries:* Repetitive strain injuries or overuse injuries occur slowly and become progressively worse over a period of time. Pain and swelling is usually of gradual onset but persists over a long period of time.

Skin and subcutaneous tissues injuries

Sharp objects, equipment or apparatus, the playing surface, etc, may cause injuries to the skin and underlying tissue. These include cuts, abrasions, infections, contusions, blisters.

When dealing with blood spill injuries, protect yourself from contact with blood. Wear rubber surgical gloves if available, or place the contact hand in a plastic bag. This is important procedure as many life-threatening viruses are transmitted through blood contamination.

Cuts

Cuts should be thoroughly cleaned and all dirt or debris removed. They should be washed or swabbed with clean water and/or antiseptic solutions, then covered with a sterile dressing. Swab from the centre outwards and use a clean area each time the wound is touched. Cover with a sterile dressing and bandage in position.

Small cuts can be covered with plasters but again clean carefully, dry and apply the gauze centre over the cut. For stab type cuts, draw the edges together with butterfly plasters. If there is extensive bleeding from a wound, cover with a sterile dressing and apply pressure with a cotton wool pad; bandage and elevate the area. Seek medical treatment as soon as possible. Large cuts over 2 cm long and gaping will require stitching – refer at once to a Casualty Department.

Abrasions

These are caused by friction or scraping of the skin, and are usually superficial. Clean and treat as cuts.

Infections

Cuts and abrasions can become infected as a result of dirt and micro-organisms penetrating the skin or hair follicles. Infections may result in boils or carbuncles which may require antibiotics to prevent them spreading to underlying tissues. Refer to a doctor if infection occurs.

Contusions

Contusion is caused by a direct blow, and results in bleeding into the tissues. Apply ice as directed over the contusion to reduce bleeding and swelling. Do not use heat or massage, as these will increase bleeding.

Blisters

Blisters are the result of pressure or friction, and prevention is better than cure. If blisters have developed, they should be left intact as the skin acts as a barrier to infection. A blister can be protected from pressure by surrounding it with a piece of plastic foam with a hole in the middle, then protected with adhesive plaster and left to heal. Large blisters or blood blisters which cause pain due to the build-up of pressure can be carefully punctured. Use a sterile needle and puncture two tiny holes in the blister. Gently squeeze out the fluid and cover with a non-adhesive sterile dressing and then plaster.

If the area is raw, clean it with water and apply an antiseptic gel or plastic skin. Use sterile equipment to avoid infection.

Muscle injuries

Injuries to muscles may be strains, partial tears or complete tears, and haematoma.

Strains

Strains will damage and result in micro tears within some fibres of the muscle. The symptoms of pain and stiffness are slow in onset and usually mild. Active movement or passive stretching will cause pain around the damaged area.

Partial tears

These result in tearing and disruption of some fibres within the muscle. The symptoms are felt immediately with severe pain and tenderness, especially when attempting to contract the muscle.

Complete tears

These involve the tearing of all muscle fibres, and the two ends of the muscle contract away from each other. Pain, swelling and tenderness is very severe and there will be complete loss of function. This type of injury may require surgery – refer quickly to hospital.

Muscular haematoma

Direct impact injuries will result in muscle rupture and bleeding. Bleeding may occur within a muscle (intramuscular) or between muscles (intermuscular). It is important to diagnose these injuries accurately as recovery from intermuscular haematoma should be relatively quick and complete. However, complications can arise following intramuscular haematoma due to intra-compartmental pressure; muscle function may be absent and recovery may be slow and incomplete.

Initially, muscle injuries should be treated with RICE as soon as possible and continued for 48–72 hours. Any vigorous movements, stretching, heat and massage must be avoided initially, as complications may result.

Tendon injuries

Tendons attach muscles to bone. Tendon injuries are either ruptures (tears) or inflammation (tendinitis).

Tears

Tendons usually tear at their weakest point, i.e. where they join the muscle at the musculo-tendinous junction. They may be *partial* tears, when some fibres are torn or *complete* tears when the tendon is severed. Pain may be mild or severe.

Complete tears may require surgery and the best results are obtained if surgery is performed immediately, before the two ends shrink and move apart. Pain is immediate, sharp and severe. It feels like a sharp blow or a 'snap' sensation in the area; the 'snap' can sometimes be heard.

Tendinitis

Inflammation of a tendon (tendinitis) and inflammation of the tendon in its sheath (tenosynovitis) are very common problems. They are usually caused by repetitive stress or overuse, but can be caused by awkward movements such as landing awkwardly or mis-hitting a ball. The pain is niggling and comes on gradually. It is worse when the tendon is moved and may progress until movements are impossible. Because the blood supply to tendons is poor, they can take a very long time to heal: up to 12 weeks or even longer.

Ligaments

Ligaments attach bone to bone; they support and stabilise joints. Ligaments are damaged when joints are forced into abnormal positions. Ligaments may be sprained, partially or completely torn.

Sprained

This occurs when a few fibres are torn, producing pain and swelling. These heal quickly with little disruption of joint movement.

Partial tears

Many fibres are torn because of greater stress. These produce severe pain and swelling, and the joint will be unstable.

Complete tears

These are very severe, producing extreme pain and swelling; the joint will be quite unstable and may dislocate. Torn ligaments may heal well without surgery but others require suturing (a stitch or stitches for closing a wound, or joining two or more structures).

Injuries to ligaments result in bruising, tenderness and swelling around the affected joint, and the healing process may take over six weeks. The joint should be supported during this time with some form of strapping. Severe tears may require a brace or plaster cast.

Menisci

These are discs of cartilage found in certain joints such as the knee, where the medial and lateral menisci lie on the upper surface of the condyles of the tibia. These may tear due to excessive forces during rotation or extreme flexion, causing acute pain and swelling. The knee may lock if a part of the discs becomes dislodged as it may interfere with the function of the knee. Surgery may be required to remove part of the cartilage but some tears heal without surgery.

Bursae

These are sacs of fluid which reduce friction between moving parts of a joint. They may lie between tendons and bones to allow smooth movement of the tendon over the bone. They usually become inflamed because of overuse or repetitive trauma.

Inflammation of a bursa is known as *bursitis*: it produces pain and swelling in the area of the bursa and radiates pain around it. It may heal with rest or may require a cortisone injection to help it settle. Very occasionally surgery is required for a chronic, persistently painful bursa.

Bone fractures

A fracture is a break in a bone. It may be classified as transverse, oblique, spiral or comminuted. Fractures may be *simple* or *compound*:

- A simple fracture is a clean break in the bone with the skin intact.
- A compound fracture involves more complex breaks of the bone and perforation of the skin.

Bones fracture due to excessive force applied to the bone. Stress or fatigue fractures occur as a result of overuse, when repetitive muscle contraction pulls on the bone. This causes repeated minor stress and damage which does not have time to heal. Fractures require immobilisation to reduce the displacement and prevent movement, thus allowing time for the fracture to heal. Fractures of the upper limb usually heal in six to eight weeks, providing there are no complications such as inadequate blood supply. However, fractures of the lower limb take 12 to 14 weeks. Fractures heal more quickly in children than adults.

Treatment of soft tissue injuries

These are general guidelines; treatment will vary depending on the type and extent of the injury. Only those with specialist knowledge should attempt to treat sports injuries.

1. *Acute phase:* for immediate treatment, apply RICED; ice applications should be used every hour and then every two to three hours.

    Slow static movements within the limit of the pain can be practised two to three times a day. These isometric movements must be performed slowly, and must stop before pain is felt. Start with three contractions only, then build up gradually to five, seven and ten, providing there is no deterioration in the condition.

2. *Sub-acute phase* (24–48 hours): continue with the above routine. Once static movements can be carried out without pain, add gentle active movements within the painfree range. When inner and middle range is pain-free, move into outer range; it is important to maintain flexibility.

No definite timescale can be set for these stages, they will depend on the extent of the injury and the speed of recovery.

Rehabilitation

Stage 1

This will begin as soon as possible after severe pain and muscle spasm eases. It is a non-weight bearing phase; ice or other modalities may be used. Free active exercises must be practised four to six times per day. Little and often is the best format – the number must increase each time. Eccentric work may be easier initially. Static stretch exercises should also be included to improve flexibility. During this phase, the unaffected parts should be exercised to maintain fitness levels, but care must be taken not to stress the injury.

Stage 2

This is a partial weight-bearing phase, which will begin when there is little swelling and no pain in nearly full range of movement. Heat can now be used, or other modalities. Muscles are exercised against light resistance with a build-up of repetitions. Partial weight-bearing exercises are practised; pain must be the guide – if it hurts, stop.

Stage 3

This is the weight-bearing phase. Strength training, flexibility and co-ordination work are included, in preparation for the return to normal activities.

Stage 4

This is a return to full function. This phase must be planned to cover all the activities that the client will encounter on return to normal situation, whether simply coping with daily living or heavy training. Much encouragement is required in this stage as movements which caused the injuries must be introduced.

It is important not to progress too quickly through each phase as injuries may recur if athletes are over anxious to return to their sport. Fitness tests must be undertaken to ensure adequate fitness levels before resuming sporting or normal activities.

Cryotherapy

Cryotherapy (cold or ice therapy) is the first line of action in the treatment of sports injury. It is effective, simple, easy to use and inexpensive. It is beneficial in the immediate (acute) post-traumatic phase, and also through the rehabilitation phases. As it is easy to apply with little danger or complication, the athlete can continue the treatment at home. Ice must be applied as soon as possible to the injured part, within 5–15 minutes. Any delay will result in secondary damage which will increase the extent of the injury. This will prolong the rate of recovery and limit the return to full normal function.

Methods of ice application

1 *Ice cubes* which are slowly moved over the area; sometimes referred to as ice massage.
2 *Crushed ice* placed in a plastic or towelling bag; place over the area with a *thin towel in between.*
3 *Gel freezer packs* which are kept frozen until required and applied to the area as above. These are convenient to use and can be refrozen and reused.
4 *Packs of frozen food* such as peas applied to the area as above; these can be refrozen and reused (but must not be eaten after defrosting).
5 *Chemical packs* which become cold when struck hard to mix the chemicals. These packs are not as effective as other methods as the temperature is not as low. There is also a danger of chemical burns, should the chemicals leak. Manufacturers are continually working on improvements.

6 *Ice-water* in a pan or bucket into which the part is immersed. Most suitable for ankle and wrist injuries. To ensure a sufficiently cold temperature, ice must float on the surface throughout the treatment.

7 *Cold aerosol sprays* are not as effective as other methods as they produce superficial cooling only. They do have the advantage of being very convenient, easy to carry around and quick to use.

Physiological effects of cooling the tissues

Certain changes will be produced in the tissues as a result of cold application – these are known as the physiological effects. These effects include:

- a decrease in metabolic rate in the area;
- a decrease in the circulation due to vasoconstriction in the area;
- local anaesthesia with a reduction in pain;
- a decrease in muscle spasm;
- a decrease in inflammatory response;
- a decrease in the flexibility of ligaments and tendons.

> **LEARN**
> Do not place ice directly on to the skin, which may result in ice burns. Always separate the ice from the skin using a towel.

Decrease in metabolic rate

This is the main reason for applying ice to the area immediately following injury. Cold reduces the metabolic rate of cells and consequently their oxygen requirement. If cold therapy is not given, the cells around the periphery of the damaged area will require oxygen to meet metabolic demands. If this demand for oxygen cannot be met because of damage to the blood vessels in the area, the cells will die. This happens within 10–15 minutes following injury and continues for around 12 hours. This will increase the amount of tissue damage and the size of the injury; it is known as 'secondary hypoxic injury'.

By decreasing the cells' metabolic rate and need for oxygen, these cells may survive until circulation is restored, thus limiting the extent of the injury.

Note: The application of heat will have the opposite effect. Heating the tissues will increase metabolic rate and the demand for oxygen, and will cause greater secondary damage. Heat must therefore *not* be used to treat immediate acute injury.

Decrease in circulation

Cold therapy produces vasoconstriction, which will reduce blood flow. Less bleeding into the tissues will facilitate quicker healing. However, the blood clotting mechanism will be activated immediately following injury; this will also prevent blood loss and will have occurred before cold packs can be applied. In addition, the constriction of capillaries in response to cold will reduce fluid exudate and tissue swelling.

Reduction of pain

Cold induces anaesthesia – the sensory receptors in the skin are inhibited and sensation is reduced but not totally absent. Initially (one minute or so after applying the ice) pain is increased. A dull radiating pain is felt which may increase for a while but will eventually pass, giving way to a prickling sensation and then numbness.

The decrease in pain will reduce the attendant muscle spasm and limit the pain-spasm-pain cycle which occurs after injury. This analgesic effect may mask the extent and seriousness of the injury, therefore the athlete or sportsperson must not return to the activity immediately following ice treatment.

Decrease in muscle spasm

It is thought that the reduction in muscle spasm is brought about by the anaesthesia, and because cold decreases nervous transmission and depresses muscle spindle sensitivity and reflex mechanisms. After injury, the body's protective mechanism increases muscle tone to prevent further damage to the tissues. Tight muscles act as a splint preventing movement and hence further damage. If this spasm is inhibited in the early stages, careful active movements can be performed, improving recovery rate. In the rehabilitative stages, less muscle spasm allows greater flexibility and increased range of movement which facilitates a speedier return to full function.

Decreased inflammatory response

It is thought that cold decreases the inflammatory response because it reduces the effects of histamine.

Decrease flexibility of ligaments and tendons

The flexibility of connective tissue decreases after cold application; ligaments and tendons are not as elastic. It is therefore important to stop cold therapy when introducing flexibility exercises. At this stage, when healing is progressing satisfactorily and there is no risk of further bleeding, some form of heat should be given. This may commence 72 hours or so after injury, but the time will depend on the rate of healing and the extent of the injury. If in doubt, continue with ice.

Uses of cryotherapy

1   Cold therapy may be used to treat soft tissue injuries in the acute, subacute, and rehabilitative stages.
2   In the acute stage, ice is applied for 15 minutes every 1–2 hours. Little and often is the best guide. It is most effective at this stage because it slows down the metabolic rate, reduces bleeding and fluid exudate thus limiting further tissue damage.
3   In the sub acute and rehabilitative stages, the time of application is increased to 20–30 minutes, 3–4 times a day. Its main use in these stages is to relieve pain and muscle spasm, and thus facilitate early active movement.
4   To treat overuse injuries.

Contra-indications
- Open bleeding wounds.
- Deficient circulation in the part.
- Lack of skin sensation.
- Hypersensitivity to cold.
- Extreme pain during application.

Factors which affect the rate of cooling

The application of cold to the area conducts heat away from the superficial and deep tissues, resulting in a decrease in temperature. There will be a rapid and immediate reduction in surface temperature, but the temperature of deeper tissues will decrease more slowly and will continue to decrease for some time after the ice is removed. There are many factors which affect the rate of cooling. These include:

1 The area of the part in contact with the ice.
2 The length of time the part is in contact with the ice.
3 The difference in temperature between the part and the ice.
4 The rate at which the body regenerates heat.
5 The rate at which heat is conducted away from the ice.

Ice packs and gel packs used for 30 minutes produce similar cooling effects, but research indicates that immersion in ice water for an equal length of time produces more intense cooling and slower rewarming. This may relate to the larger surface area being treated.

Chemical packs are less effective at reducing temperature than the other methods, and cold sprays produce superficial, temporary cooling only.

Treatment

Remember the RICE routine (rest, ice, compression, elevation).

Ice must be applied as soon as possible, within 5–10 minutes of the injury occurring. Immediate appropriate treatment will increase effectiveness and considerably shorten the recovery period. Ice should be applied as soon as an initial assessment of the injury has been made.

The method of application will depend on availability and convenience. Chipped or crushed ice in a bag, gel packs from a refrigerator, or ice cubes are suitable for most injuries; ice water in a bucket or bowl is suitable for ankle, calf, wrist, forearm and elbow injuries.

If ice is placed in direct contact with the skin it can stick and long-term application can produce ice burns. It is therefore essential to oil the skin lightly before stroking with an ice cube, and to place a thin layer of cold wet towel or bandage on the skin when using an ice pack, i.e. between the skin and the ice pack. The part may be immersed in iced water without protection, but if pain is intense the part must be removed from the water for 15–30 seconds and then reimmersed.

Rest is important, as any movement may produce further damage increasing the extent of the injury. Compression may be applied and the part elevated if possible to assist drainage.

Technique using ice pack or gel pack

1   Prepare the ice pack by placing approximately 1 kg of crushed ice in a plastic or towelling bag; alternatively, pile the ice onto the towel and fold the ends over. If using a cold pack, remove from the freezer just before use.
2   Ensure that the client is comfortable, well supported and in a suitable position to receive the treatment.
3   Remove any clothing or jewellery from the area.
4   Explain the treatment to the client, highlighting the beneficial effects and the importance of regular timed application. Explain that pain may be felt or increase initially, but that this will give way to pins and needles and then numbness. If pain continues remove the ice.
5   Wring out a towel in cold or iced water and place over the injured part. Place the cold pack over this and wrap a double layer of towelling around the part to hold the pack in place. If intense pain develops, the ice must be removed for 15–30 seconds and then reapplied.
6   Compression should be applied and the part elevated and rested.
7   Treat for 15 minutes initially, increasing to 30 minutes in the subacute stage, but this will depend on client tolerance. Pale skin should be red, dark skin will be darker.
8   Repeat the procedure every two hours for the first 24 hours after injury, or as often as possible.
9   Exercise as explained below.

Technique using iced water

1   Fill the container to three-quarters full with cold water and ice. Ensure that there is ice floating in the water throughout the treatment.
2   Position the client in a comfortable position; remove all clothing and jewellery around the injury.
3   Explain the treatment to the client as in point 4 above.
4   Immerse the part in the water and reassure that pain is to be expected initially but that it will subside. If the pain is intolerable, lift the part out of the water for 15–30 seconds then reimmerse.
5   Keep immersing the part until it is numb and red; aim for 20 minutes.
6   Remove the part from the water and dry gently.
7   Exercise as explained below.

Technique with ice cube massage

1   Place a supply of ice cubes in a container.
2   Position the client in a comfortable, well-supported position; elevate the part if possible.
3   Remove all clothing and jewellery from the area.
4   Explain the procedure to the client.
5   Spread a thin layer of oil over the area.
6   Hold the ice cube with folded tissue or lint.

7 Move the ice slowly over the part, moving up and down in straight lines; overlap the previous stroke. Work over and around the injured part. The ice will melt, so ensure that there is a towel under the part to absorb the water.

8 Continue working in this way for 20 minutes or so, until the part is red and numb.

9 Dry the area gently.

10 Exercise as explained below.

Technique with cold sprays

These aerosol sprays are not as effective as other methods, and are generally used for convenience on the field of play. The part is uncovered and sprayed at a certain distance for a few seconds. It is important that these sprays are used according to manufacturer's directions, as their mode of application may vary. If incorrectly applied they can cause ice burns.

Exercises following cryotherapy

During the first 24–48 hours, ice application is followed by slow, gentle *isometric* exercises. These static muscle contractions are performed within the pain-free range.

As healing progresses, *isotonic* movements are performed. The client is instructed to move the joint slowly through to the point just before pain is felt, to hold for a moment and return. All possible joint movements must be practised in this way. Great care must be taken during this sub-acute stage since movement can disturb the healing process and increase secondary damage.

Remember: movements must not produce pain. All movements must be within the limit of pain.

Example: Treatment to injured ankle joint, where injuries are usually to the lateral or medial ligaments.

- Apply cold therapy for up to 30 minutes, then remove.
- Static exercise instruction – 'I'm going to hold your foot firmly and I want you to pull as hard as you can against my hand, stop if there is any pain'. The resistance against the movement must be even, and great enough to produce tension within the muscle but to prevent any movement. Initially the resistance is applied to dorsi flexion (hand applying resistance on the dorsum of the foot), and is then applied to plantar flexion (hand on the sole of the foot). When these contractions are easy to perform, inversion and eversion are added. Exercise away from the injury first, i.e. for lateral ligament injury, perform static inversion first. When this is easy, carefully perform static eversion (this may not be possible initially). Each contraction is held for five to six seconds.
  Remember: tension must be developed within the pain-free limit.
- After 48–72 hours or so, depending on the severity of the injury, ice treatment is followed by isotonic exercises.
- Instruction for isotonic movement – 'Pull the foot up slowly towards you (dorsi flexion); stop when you feel any pain; hold; now move the foot slowly down away from you.' (plantar flexion). Repeat for inversion and eversion and then progress to circumduction. Perform three movements of each initially, increasing by two with each application.

Practice Tasks

Explain how and why you would teach a client to breathe correctly (refer to page 42):

Devise a record card that you would use during the initial consultation and assessment of each client, prior to their exercise classes (refer to chapter 13):

Study a variety of exercise videos, exercise books and magazine articles and complete the following tasks.

List any exercises that you would consider unsafe:

Devise your own set of warm-up exercises:

Devise a set of aerobic exercises:

Devise a set of cool-down exercises:

QUESTIONS

1. List the methods by which ice may be applied.
2. Discuss the physiological effects of cooling the tissues.
3. List the contra-indications to cold therapy.
4. List the factors which affect the rate of cooling.
5. Explain the importance of applying oil to the skin prior to ice massage.
6. State how frequently ice should be administered during the first 24 hours.

References and further reading

Alter, Michael J. (1988). *Science of Sketching*, Human Kinetics Books. An excellent book for anyone requiring any information on flexibility work.

American Council on Exercise (1991). *Aerobic Dance-Exercise Instructors Manual*. A useful source of detailed information for anyone leading aerobic classes.

Beashel, Paul, and Taylor, John (1988) *Sport Examined*, Macmillan Education.

Cross, Gibbs and Gray (1991), *The Sporting Body*, Sydney: McGraw Hill Book Co.

Curzon, L.B. (1976), *Teaching in Further Education*, London: Cassell.

Daniels, Lucille, and Worthington, Catherine (1977), *Therapeutic Exercise*, WB Saunders Co. Comprehensive information on correct and maintenance of posture and body alignment.

Davies, Kimmel and Anly (1988), *Physical Education Theory & Practice*, Macmillan Company (Australia). Covers the detail of exercise theory. Interesting additional reading.

Grisogono, Vivian (1984), *Sports Injuries*, London: John Murray. A good self-help guide on the avoidance and treatment of sports injuries.

Hazeldine, R. (1993). *Fitness for Sport*, The Crowood Press. Excellent, clearly explained information for individuals training for or teaching the theory of fitness. Good examples of exercise programmes, circuits, etc., for achieving set goals.

Kennedy, Legel and Sagamore (1992), *Anatomy of an Exercise Class*, Human Kinetics Books. Gives detailed information on the degrees of movement possible at body joints. Excellent information on analysis of exercises.

Luby, Sue, and St Onge, Richard A. (1986), *Body Sense*, Faber & Faber Inc. A well-illustrated book clearly showing the hazards of poor postural alignment. Covers the fundamentals of breathing, posture and alignment, stretching techniques and other useful topics.

Sharkey, B.J. (1990), *Physiology of Fitness*, Human Kinetics Books. Gives detailed information on the physiological aspects of exercise.

Smith, B. (1993), *Advanced Fitness Teachers Manual*, Ludoe Publications (Loughborough University). Gives specific information on training for the components of fitness.

St George, Francine (1990), *The Muscle Fitness Book*, The Crowood Press. Good guidelines on safe, effective exercise for specific sporting activities.

Time-Life Books (1990), *Cross Training – Ultimate Fitness*. Interesting reading for those interested in the concept of cross training. A good chapter on 'Eating for Performance' gives recipes for suitable foods.

Index